Help4ADD@HighSchool

The book you'll want to read
even if your mom
bought it for you! :-)

by Kathleen G. Nadeau, Ph.D.

Published by Advantage Books
8607 Cedar St.
Silver Spring, MD 20910

Nadeau, Kathleen G.
    Help4ADD@highschool / by Kathleen G. Nadeau
        p.   cm.
    Includes bibliographical references.
    ISBN 0-9660366-1-1
    1. Attention-deficit-disordered youth—Education (Secondary)—
    United States—Handbooks, manuals, etc.—Juvenile literature.
    I. Title: Help4ADD@HighSchool
    LC4713.4.N33   1998   98-8578
                                                                      CIP
                                                                       AC

10 9 8 7 6 5 4 3
Printed in the U.S.A.

Dedication

This book is dedicated to my daughter, Langdon, whose high school years were filled with challenges, in the hope that high schools can become more responsive to the needs of students with ADD.

Acknowledgements

I would like to acknowledge the help of many high school students who have shared their hopes, their frustrations, and their struggles with me as they worked their way through the four most difficult academic years for students with ADD. I would especially like to thank Kerith Hartmann, Mara Whitney and Patrick Quinn for taking time to read drafts of my book and to offer very helpful insight. I would also like to thank Barbara Michaluk for her never flagging support of this project through the many pitfalls we encountered along the way, and Sam Carter, who worked beyond the call of duty to create his illustrations for this book.

Illustrator

This book was illustrated by Sam Carter, a 17-year-old cartoonist from Carrollton, GA. Upon graduating from Carrollton High School, Sam hopes to attend the Savannah College of Art and Design, where he plans to study film and sequential art.

Learn

Improve
Grades

Graduate

Get a Life

B Happy

Find Talents

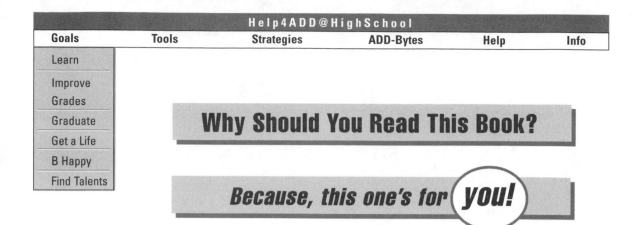

Why Should You Read This Book?

Because, this one's for you!

Help4ADD@HighSchool won't lecture you, nag you, or tell you that you'll spend the rest of your life in a McJob if you don't study.

It **WILL** help you to figure out: how to find your groove; how to make your life in high school more ADD-Friendly; how to survive and thrive in high school with ADD; and how to get ready for life after school.

Help4ADD@HighSchool is written as a series of short topics that can be read one at a time if you want. The topics are clustered into sections—like "school," "family," or "friends," so you can easily find what you're looking for.

This book is written to help YOU learn how to take charge of your ADD : . .

◆ so that you can have the kind of future you want

◆ so that you can feel excited about your future

◆ so that you can do more than just count the days until high school ends.

Help4ADD@HighSchool is written to be ADD Friendly

Help4ADD@HighSchool is written to be readable and **ADD-Friendly**. By "ADD-Friendly," we mean a book that is easy to read for someone with ADD. If you lose concentration easily, just pick out topics that interest you and skip the rest. You don't have to read long, boring chapters to get the answer you're looking for. This book is written to be readable, interesting, and fun!

Read more about making things **"ADD-Friendly"** as you go through this book.

Help4ADD@HighSchool

. . . is ADD-Friendly because it's:

- ◆ easy to read
- ◆ written in -"bytes"
- ◆ laid out in an "open" page format.

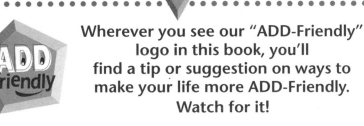

Wherever you see our "ADD-Friendly" logo in this book, you'll find a tip or suggestion on ways to make your life more ADD-Friendly. Watch for it!

Other books by Kathleen Nadeau

Learning to Slow Down and Pay Attention, $9.95
>   with Ellen Dixon
>   A book for elementary school-aged children that explains ADD
>   in kid-friendly terms.

A College Survival Guide for Students with ADD and LD, $9.95
>   Tips and strategies for surviving and thriving in college.
>   Brief, practical, and highly readable.

Adventures in Fast Forward, $18.95
>   Practical approaches for adults on how to take charge of their ADD.

ADD in the Workplace, $23.95
>   Career choices, changes, and challenges for adults with ADD.

A Comprehensive Guide to ADD in Adults, $39.95
>   Edited by Kathleen G. Nadeau, Ph.D.
>   A book for professionals, and for those who want a more in-depth
>   understanding of ADD in adults.

>   All of these books can be ordered by calling Advantage Books,
>   Toll free: 1-888-238-8588.

HOME PAGE

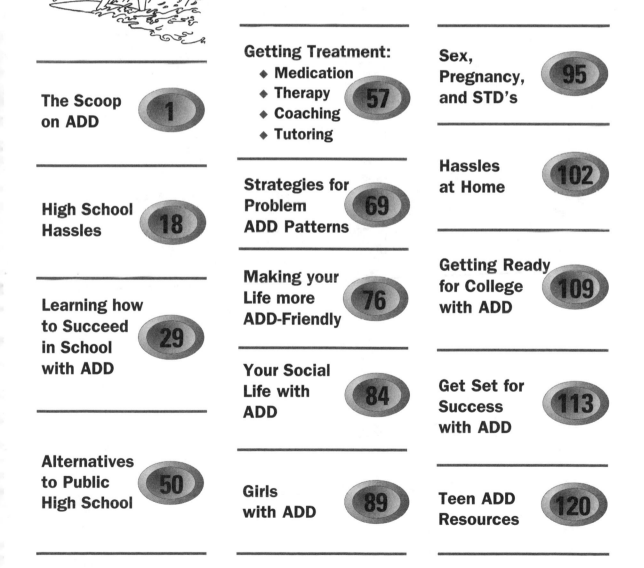

"Surf" this book! Here's how:

Check out this home page to see what awaits you. Go to the "hot buttons" beside each topic and flip to the section that covers what you're looking for. Tabs on right-hand pages let you quickly "surf" from section to section.

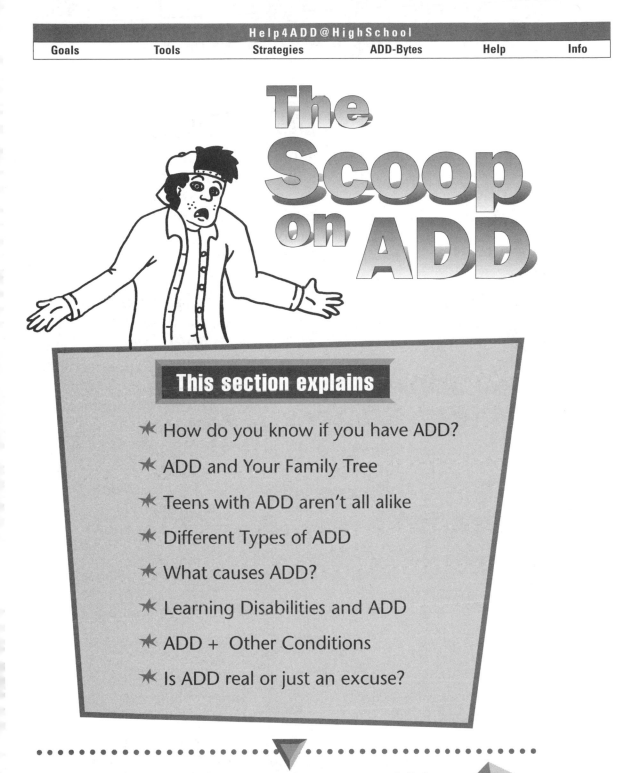

The Scoop on ADD

This section explains

✳ How do you know if you have ADD?

✳ ADD and Your Family Tree

✳ Teens with ADD aren't all alike

✳ Different Types of ADD

✳ What causes ADD?

✳ Learning Disabilities and ADD

✳ ADD + Other Conditions

✳ Is ADD real or just an excuse?

Even if you were diagnosed with ADD as a child and think you know all about it, it might help to read this section. ADD doesn't just mean "hyper" or "short attention span." The more you know about ADD, the better you'll be able to manage it.

ADD Friendly

1

ADD and your family tree

ADD is something that "runs" in families. If you have ADD, it's very likely that you're not the only one in the family who does. That doesn't mean that someone else has actually been diagnosed with ADD. There are many adults with ADD who have never been diagnosed, because we've begun only recently to understand and recognize ADD in adults.

It is likely if you have ADD, that one of your parents may show some ADD-like patterns, or that you have aunts and uncles who have ADD traits.

What would these traits look like? You may have a relative who seems smart, but who dropped out of school before graduating. This was a common pattern for people with ADD who never got any help. They may be really active and on-the-go; they may be forgetful and disorganized; or really messy. They may start a lot of projects they never seem to finish, or have piles of papers and magazines they never throw away. They may always run late. These are a few patterns that are common in adults with ADD.

You may be the ADD pioneer in your family, the first one to be diagnosed and to learn what to do about your ADD.

That will be good for you, and may even help other people in your family who haven't gotten help for their ADD symptoms.

After you read this book, you can share what you've learned. **It works a lot better if your whole family becomes "ADD-smart."** Then you can get along more smoothly at home, and know how to support each other at school, at work, and in reaching goals.

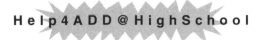

Teens with ADD aren't all alike

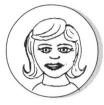

Marie, a junior in high school, is quiet and shy. She seldom talks to classmates. Marie often feels lost during class, but is afraid to embarrass herself by asking questions. At night, she really struggles with homework. It takes her hours. Even when she studies hard for tests she "blanks out" during exams.

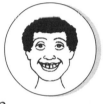

Mark is a top soccer player. He loves to hang around his soccer buddies, and is never happier than when he is talking, moving, and playing sports. In class he feels bored and sleepy. He usually tries to cram in homework during homeroom or when he's on the bus. After soccer practice, the last thing he feels like doing is homework at night.

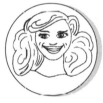

Sandy is a ball of energy. With her long, curly hair, and dark eyes, she has a very dramatic look, which she emphasizes with black eyeliner and deep red lipstick. Sandy talks a mile-a-minute and loves to hang out with her theater friends. In class, she loves to debate with the teacher and does pretty well on tests, but her grades are low because she rarely does homework assignments. Theater productions at school are what she lives for. Sandy dreams of going to New York one day to become an actress.

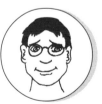

Steve, a gifted student, spends hours in front of his computer. He works hard to earn good grades and hopes to go to a top college. He never seems to have any free time. Between homework and extra-curricular activities, he's often working until mid-night and wakes up tired most school mornings. He has to take careful notes when he reads. Otherwise he forgets everything. Writing papers is a huge struggle. He has good ideas—in fact too many good ideas. They all get tangled in his head, and he has trouble untangling them to get them down on paper.

As different as these four high school students may seem, they all have ADD.

Surprised?

3

Different types of ADD

You probably know people who have ADD because it's a common problem. People who are really hyperactive and seem to run 90 miles per hour all the time are easy to spot. But not everyone with ADD is "hyper". Some teens with ADD are day-dreamers or couch potatoes!

People with ADD share some traits, like having trouble concentrating, being absent-minded or disorganized, but they're all unique, with their own personalities, their own skills, and interests.

You can have ADD a little or a lot. Some people are only mildly affected by ADD while others are VERY affected.

There are three main "types" of ADD

1.	The first type is the **"hyperactive/impulsive type"** that most people know about.
2.	The second type is called **"inattentive type."** Someone who has "inattentive type" ADD, may be calm and quiet, but has trouble remembering, organizing, getting things done, and staying tuned in. They may seem a little "spacey," or tend to day-dream in class. More girls seem to have this kind of ADD than the "hyper" kind.
3.	The third type is called **"combined type,"** which means that they have both hyperactive and inattentive tendencies. This is probably the most common type of ADD.

Which type do you think you might have?

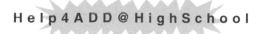
What causes ADD?

ADD is something you are born with. Doctors and scientists don't understand everything about ADD, but we have lots of evidence that ADD is inherited. ADD brains don't have enough of a neurochemical called Dopamine, so certain parts of the brain that help us to: pay attention, control our impulses, stick with a plan, organize, remember what we need to do, sit still, focus, and concentrate don't work as well as they should all the time. Stimulant medications help increase the supply of Dopamine in our brains.

THE SCOOP ON ADD

Learning Disabilities and ADD

Learning disabilities are very common in people with ADD. That doesn't necessarily mean that you have been diagnosed with learning disabilities in school—schools have their own definitions of LD. But if you have ADD, you may also have difficulty with things like:

- ◆ Recalling information
- ◆ Remembering names
- ◆ Organizing your thoughts
- ◆ Remembering math facts
- ◆ Learning a foreign language
- ◆ Spelling and grammar
- ◆ Accidentally leaving out words or phrases when you write.

ADD Friendly

If you have any of these types of learning difficulties, you may want to have an evaluation for learning problems. Even if you don't qualify for LD services in high school, or don't WANT these kinds of support services, it could still help to be evaluated if you plan to go on to college. LD support services for college students with learning problems are really different from high school. You are not singled out, labeled, or embarrassed, and there are many supports that can help you be much more successful in college.

5

ADD+

ADD plus other conditions

ADD is often found in combination with other conditions. These other conditions seem to come in "clusters" and seem to "run" in families just like ADD does.

It's important that you have a complete evaluation conducted by someone who is expert not only in ADD, but also in these coexisting conditions. If you have a coexisting condition, it won't do much good to focus only on your ADD and ignore whatever else is going on. You're a complex person who happens to have ADD. We need to consider ALL of you, not just your ADD.

What are some of the conditions that commonly coexist with ADD?

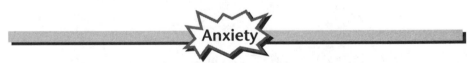
Anxiety

If you suffer from ADD+ anxiety, chances are you feel worried or tense a lot of the time. You may have trouble relaxing and falling asleep at night. Stimulant medication for ADD may make you feel even more tense unless you also take medication to reduce your anxiety.

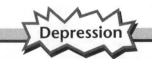
Depression

It is very common to experience ADD+ depression. More girls with ADD than boys seem to suffer from depression. You may feel overwhelmed by school, and by all the things you're trying to keep up with. Teens who are depressed may feel tired, irritable, negative, and discouraged. Don't confuse depression with feeling "down" for a few days because something has disappointed you. Depression can last for weeks and sometimes months.

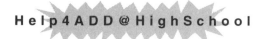
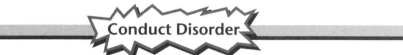

Conduct Disorder

More guys than girls are likely to have a conduct disorder. Kids who often lose their temper, are very argumentative, are defiant, and deliberately do things to annoy people, sometimes become teens with Conduct Disorder. Conduct-disordered teens may skip school, run away from home, act aggressively, and engage in vandalism. Teenagers with ADD+ conduct disorder are at risk for ending up in trouble with the law.

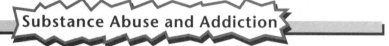

Substance Abuse and Addiction

Teens with ADD often are more impulsive, and more likely to take risks that may lead into drug and alcohol experimentation at a young age. Teens with undiagnosed ADD may be drawn to marijuana, alcohol, or cocaine in an attempt to self-medicate their ADD. Teens with ADD are at higher risk for addiction.

THE SCOOP ON ADD

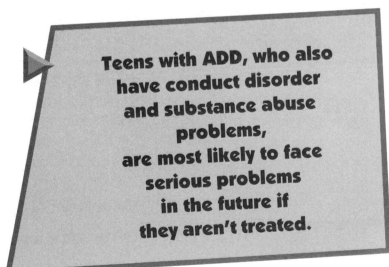

Teens with ADD, who also have conduct disorder and substance abuse problems, are most likely to face serious problems in the future if they aren't treated.

Learning Disabilities and ADD

We've already mentioned that LD and ADD are often found together. In fact, there are some experts who believe that everyone with ADD also has some other type of learning disorder. If you do have other learning difficulties, they will not be helped by medication. You may mistakenly think that the stimulant medication "doesn't help" your ADD when it's really a learning problem that has been unidentified. It's important to understand the differences between problems that medication helps, and learning problems that need a tutor's help.

Don't worry

Don't worry, or let this list of **ADD+** conditions discourage you. Many teens with ADD don't have other conditions, and even those who do can be treated very successfully.

Do worry

Do worry, if you're involved in substance abuse, antisocial, or illegal activity! Those are serious problems that you need to tackle before they get worse.

Is ADD Real?

You may meet people who don't "believe" in ADD. They think ADD is just an excuse for being lazy, for not trying, or for being irresponsible. People who make these remarks are only showing their ignorance of ADD.

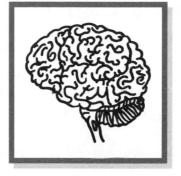

We now have new kinds of medical tests that measure activity in our brains—like how much blood is flowing in certain areas, or how much fuel is being used by different parts. By taking special pictures of the brain with brain-imaging techniques, we can see very real differences between brains of people with ADD and with those who don't have ADD. People who say that ADD isn't real don't know what they're talking about!

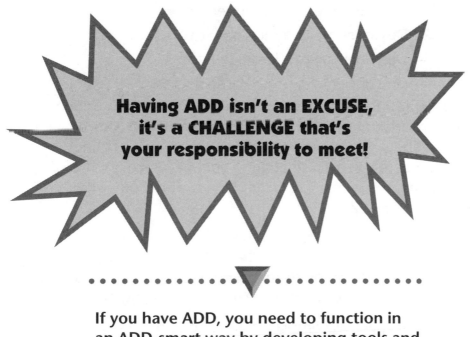

Having ADD isn't an EXCUSE, it's a CHALLENGE that's your responsibility to meet!

If you have ADD, you need to function in an ADD-smart way by developing tools and strategies to meet the challenges of ADD.

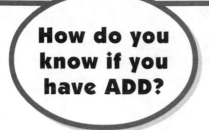

How do you know if you have ADD?

To get an accurate diagnosis for ADD, you need to see a professional with expertise in ADD. He or she can evaluate you for ADD, and also for any of the ADD+ symptoms that need to be treated along with your ADD.

We have included below a questionnaire for teens who think they might have ADD. If you answer with a 3 or 4 to many questions, then it's probably a good idea to get an evaluation for ADD.

 High School ADD Questionnaire

Rate EVERY statement by placing the appropriate number that most fits you in the space to the left of each item. If an item does not apply to you, just write NA.

    0—Does not describe me at all

    1—Describes me to a slight degree

    2—Describes me to a moderate degree

    3—Describes me to a large degree

    4—Describes me to a very large degree

Please feel free to make comments in the margins or on the space provided at the end of each question sheet. Our goal is to find out about you, so it's important that you tell us things like, "This is true to a very large degree, but only when I'm tired." Or, "Sometimes this is true to a large degree, but at other times it's not a problem at all."

Inattention

_____ It's hard for me to stick with one thing for a long time (except TV, computer games, or hanging out).

_____ My parents complain that I often don't listen when they talk to me.

_____ I tune in and out when I'm in class.

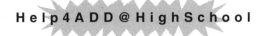

_____ It's hard for me to study for long periods of time.

_____ When I read, my eyes scan the words, but my mind is somewhere else.

_____ I often miss the teacher's instructions because I'm not listening.

Impulsivity

_____ I "get in trouble" at school for doing minor things.

_____ I usually "go with my feelings" instead of thinking things out.

_____ I have a habit of interrupting when I'm talking to people.

_____ Sometimes I say things without meaning to.

_____ I like to do things when the mood hits me.

_____ I make snap decisions.

_____ Following directions is frustrating; I'd rather dive in and figure things out as I go.

_____ Sometimes I create problems because I do things without thinking about the consequences.

Hyperactivity

_____ My friends say I'm "hyper."

_____ I often jiggle, or fiddle with something.

_____ I feel restless sitting in class.

_____ I feel tired when I have to sit still in class, but have energy when I'm moving between classes.

_____ I'm a lot calmer if I play sports or exercise every day.

_____ I talk a lot.

_____ It's hard for me to chill out and relax.

THE SCOOP ON ADD

Distractibility

_____ I daydream in class.

_____ Even when I try to listen to the teacher, my thoughts wander.

_____ I dread being called on in class, because I'm usually tuned out and don't hear the question.

_____ I am easily distracted from my work when other students are talking.

_____ Friends tease me about being spacey.

_____ I need to play the radio when I study so that I can concentrate.

_____ I look around in class when I'm supposed to be looking at the teacher.

Hyperfocusing

_____ Sometimes I'm so "into" doing something, that I don't hear people call me.

_____ I can get totally lost in doing something and lose track of time.

_____ It's hard for me to stop doing something I'm really involved in when it's time to shift to a new activity.

Organization

_____ I have trouble planning a long paper or a big project.

_____ I have trouble organizing my ideas when I try to write.

_____ Projects and papers are hard for me to complete.

_____ My backpack is totally disorganized.

_____ My desk is really messy.

_____ My room is a disaster area.

_____ I have trouble getting ready and organized for school in the morning.

Memory/Forgetfulness

_____ I forget to bring home papers and permission slips.

_____ I forget to do what people ask me to do.

_____ I forget to take things to school that I'll need later.

_____ I forget to bring home the books I need for homework.

_____ I forget my homework assignments.

_____ I often forget appointments.

_____ I often lose my keys.

_____ If I don't write things down I'll forget them.

_____ I'm always forgetting where I left my stuff.

_____ My mom or dad have to constantly remind me of things.

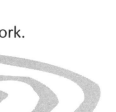

Perseverance

_____ I give up on things when I feel frustrated.

_____ I start hobbies and projects but don't finish them.

_____ I get bored with lessons or other activities that require practice and usually quit doing them.

_____ I only do the things that come easy to me; I rarely stick with something long enough to develop a skill or talent.

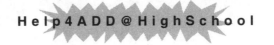
Self-discipline

_____ I have been called lazy.

_____ I have been called irresponsible.

_____ I have trouble staying motivated.

_____ I never make resolutions because I know I won't keep them.

_____ I usually do what I like to do instead of what I ought to do.

Time-management

_____ I don't wear a watch and don't like to keep track of the time.

_____ I am a procrastinator.

_____ I am often late.

_____ I usually underestimate how long things will take me.

_____ I keep people waiting.

_____ I often get home after my curfew because I lose track of time.

_____ I often miss the bus.

Academics

_____ I have been called an underachiever.

_____ My parents and teachers tell me I need to try harder.

_____ My grades are pulled down because I usually don't do my homework.

_____ I have trouble finishing assignments in class.

_____ I am worried about school.

_____ I'm afraid I won't get into college.

_____ I turn in assignments late.

_____ I can't stand school and can't wait to graduate.

_____ My grades vary from "A's" to "F's."

_____ Sometimes I study for a test, but then I "blank out" on the exam.

_____ My grades are lowered by careless errors.

Frustration tolerance

_____ I hate to wait.

_____ People tell me I'm impatient.

_____ I lose my temper pretty easily when I'm frustrated.

_____ I have hit, kicked, or broken things when I felt frustrated.

_____ I tend to quit doing things that frustrate me, even if they are important.

_____ When I don't understand my homework, I usually quit trying.

Temper/Aggression

_____ I lose my temper or argue frequently.

_____ I have a short fuse.

_____ It's impossible for me to stay cool if someone is mad or yelling at me.

_____ I've gotten into fights at school because I've lost my temper.

15

_____ When someone teases or taunts me I become aggressive.

_____ I hit or shove when I'm angry.

_____ Coaches have warned me not to be so aggressive during a game.

_____ I have frequent physical fights with a brother, sister, or classmate.

_____ I have been so angry that I've cursed at my mom or dad.

_____ I have driven dangerously or too fast because I was angry.

Feelings about myself

_____ I feel embarrassed because I don't know what I'm supposed to do in class.

_____ I feel shy or timid around my classmates.

_____ I get upset more easily than my friends.

_____ I often feel bad about myself.

_____ I hate to be in competitive situations.

_____ No matter how hard I try, I never seem to get things right.

_____ I feel really discouraged about school and about my future.

_____ Sometimes I feel anxious and overwhelmed by all of the things that I'm supposed to do.

_____ I have frequent headaches.

_____ I have frequent stomachaches.

_____ Sometimes I exaggerate how sick I feel just so I can stay home from school.

Relationships with Adults

_____ I feel criticized by my mom.

_____ I feel criticized by my dad.

_____ I wish my parents and teachers knew how hard I try.

_____ I wish everyone would get off my back.

_____ I wish I didn't fight and argue so much with my parents.

This questionnaire has asked you about a lot of problems and issues that are typical for teens with ADD. There are plenty of teens without ADD who have many of these same problems. If you find that you answered with 3's or 4's to many questions, you should talk to an expert on ADD—a doctor or psychologist—so that they can tell you if you really have ADD, and help you find solutions for these problems. In fact, this book is full of solutions to all kinds of ADD problems. So get going, good luck, and don't feel you have to tackle it alone!

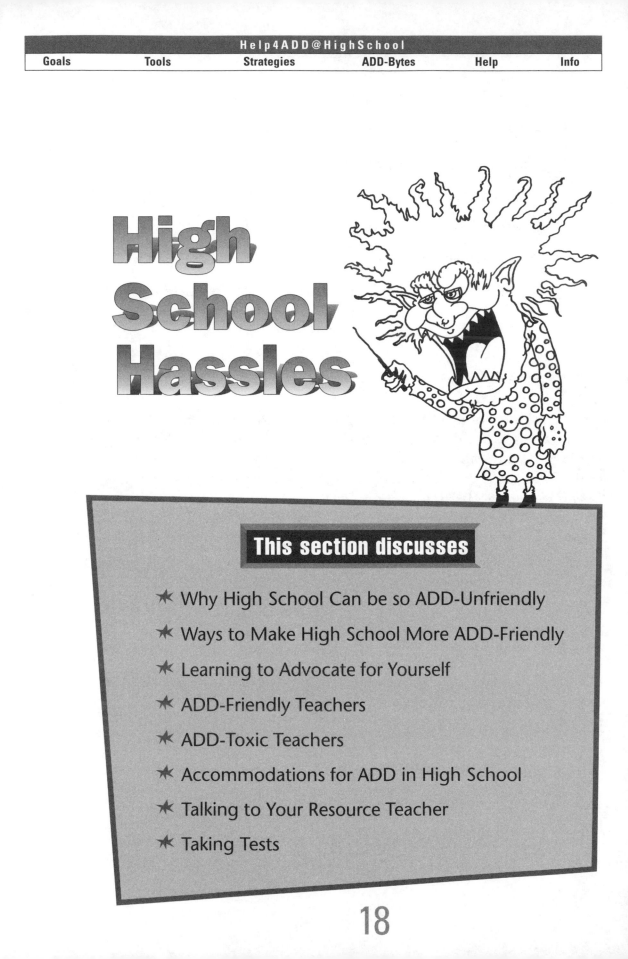

High School Hassles

This section discusses

* Why High School Can be so ADD-Unfriendly

* Ways to Make High School More ADD-Friendly

* Learning to Advocate for Yourself

* ADD-Friendly Teachers

* ADD-Toxic Teachers

* Accommodations for ADD in High School

* Talking to Your Resource Teacher

* Taking Tests

**HIGH SCHOOL YEARS
CAN BE SOME
OF THE MOST
"ADD-UN-FRIENDLY"
YEARS OF YOUR LIFE!**

**LET'S TAKE A
LOOK AT WHY . . .**

◆ **Fatigue**
high school starts too
early in the morning

◆ **Boredom**
forced to take classes
you're not interested in

◆ **Day is too long**
impossible to concen-
trate for seven periods

◆ **Too much homework**
can't work all day and at night too

◆ **Have to sit still**
even when you feel restless

◆ **Too much listening**
not enough action and interaction

◆ **Your day is controlled**
Can't take a break when you need to

◆ **Distracting**
hard to concentrate in noise and confusion

◆ **Too many rules**
very little independence or freedom

◆ **Not enough high-interest activities**
if you don't keep your grades up, you can't do the extracurricular things you like

◆ **Too many things to keep track of**
notes, assignments, and projects for six or seven classes

HIGH SCHOOL HASSLES

WAYS TO MAKE HIGH SCHOOL MORE . . .

ADD Friendly

Think about the list of why high school is often ADD-Unfriendly, and use your ADD creativity to think of some solutions. High school may never be your ideal environment, but there are things you can do to make it better!

Fighting the fatigue factor

◆ Try to get to bed earlier at night (see section on sleep problems, p. 73).

◆ Pay attention to your "best" times of day, and take your hardest classes at these times. If you feel half-asleep when you get to school in the morning, don't sign up for your most difficult classes during first or second periods.

Fighting the boredom factor

◆ Try to sign up for the most interesting teachers.

◆ Get involved in class. Passively sitting for hours is much more boring than talking, asking questions, and discussing ideas.

Fighting distractibility

◆ Sit up front and in the center of class if you can. You'll be less distracted by other students and more involved.

◆ Take notes while the teacher is talking—this will help you maintain concentration.

Dealing with restlessness

◆ Keep something with you to fiddle with—something small that makes no noise—but don't let yourself be tempted to toss it to a friend or your "help" will become a "hindrance."

◆ Get regular, daily exercise.

◆ Try to arrange your schedule so that you have periods of activity interspersed throughout the day—lunch, PE, art or shop, chorus, band, etc.

Coping with homework

◆ Do homework in small bits—on the bus, before class, when you first get home, just after dinner. Dividing homework into small bits is easier than sitting down to a two-or-three-hour stretch in the evening.

◆ Get a tutor to teach you how to write and study more efficiently—many people with ADD take far too long on homework because they haven't learned effective study techniques.

◆ Get help getting organized—an assignment book; a folder in your backpack for daily assignments; a large calendar above your desk at home so that you can visually plan long-term projects.

HIGH SCHOOL HASSLES

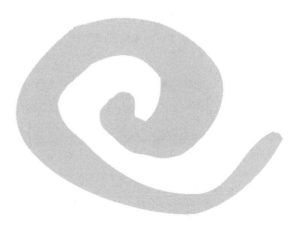

21

More tips to make High School years ADD-Friendly

With the help of your resource teacher or guidance counselor, there are other things you can do to make high school more "ADD-Friendly."

◆ **Work closely with your academic advisor**

to choose courses each semester.

◆ **Customize your registration**.

Ask for customized registration rather than computerized registration. This will let you carefully choose the best periods to take your most difficult subjects. Take them at times of day when your energy is highest.

◆ **Work hard to develop a good relationship with your teachers.**

Teachers usually work hard to help students who are involved and motivated. Try to problem-solve with your teacher. Don't wait until there is a problem before talking to your teacher about your ADD. Let your teacher know that you're trying.

◆ **Summer school**

Consider taking (or auditing) a really tough course in summer school. You can concentrate on it without all of the competing courses and activities of the school year.

◆ **Community College**

Explore taking courses at the community college for high school credit. Sometimes college courses are more interesting and challenging and often can be taken in summer school.

◆ **Work with an ADD Tutor or Coach**

A tutor or coach, who specializes in students with ADD, can teach you all kinds of tips and strategies to overcome procrastination, to become more organized, and to study more efficiently.

Learning to Advocate for Yourself in School

If you were diagnosed with ADD as a kid, chances are your mom or dad talked with your teacher several times each year, trying to find ways to help you learn and get better grades.

Your ADD probably concerned your parents more than it concerned you. They were your "advocates" with the school system.

You're in high school now, and it's time for you to learn to "advocate" for yourself.

Advocate means knowing:

- ◆ exactly how YOU are affected by ADD
- ◆ how to explain your ADD to your teachers
- ◆ exactly what to ask for from your teachers
- ◆ how to demonstrate that you are motivated and not just asking for "unfair" advantages
- ◆ how to avoid using your ADD as an excuse.

Practice Your Advocacy Skills!

If you're used to your parents fighting for you, it'll take practice to learn to stand up for yourself. You'll meet teachers and other people—maybe coaches and even counselors—"who don't believe" in ADD.

- ◆ Learn to talk comfortably about your ADD. Practice with someone you feel comfortable with—a counselor, a parent, a therapist, a friend. Learn to explain your ADD and how it affects you in class.

- ◆ Advocate for yourself *BEFORE PROBLEMS BEGIN*—talk to each teacher at the start of each term. Don't wait until you are behind on a paper or have just earned a bad grade on a test!

- ◆ Show your teacher that you are motivated. If you bombed a test, ask if there is something you can do for extra-credit to make up for the bad grade.

- ◆ Form a good relationship with your academic counselor. If you have a teacher who responds very negatively to you in the beginning of the term, try to transfer to another section of the course after discussing this with your counselor.

HIGH SCHOOL HASSLES

ADD Friendly

ADD-Friendly Teachers

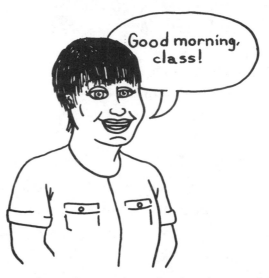

Good morning, class!

There are plenty of terrific teachers for students with ADD. How do you spot one?

- ◆ A teacher who is excited about a subject, and works in creative ways to get you excited too.

- ◆ A teacher who is flexible, and tries to work with you instead of rigidly sticking to "the rules."

- ◆ A teacher who encourages rather than lectures when you're having difficulties.

- ◆ A teacher who understands that ADD can cause forgetfulness even when you're really trying to remember.

- ◆ A teacher who is organized and clear about what is required in the course.

- ◆ A teacher who is fun and interesting, and seems to enjoy the class.

Take time to look for terrific teachers in your school! It's worth the effort. Most students with ADD do much better in the classes of teachers whom they like.

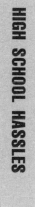

"ADD-Toxic" Teachers!

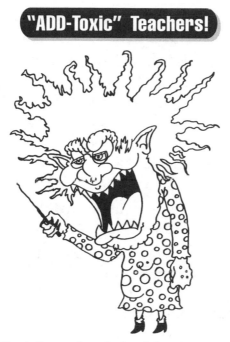

An "ADD-Toxic" teacher is bad for you and your ADD. Examples of "toxic" teachers are:

◆ A teacher who doesn't "believe in" ADD, and refuses to accommodate you.

◆ A teacher who shows little interest in his/ her students.

◆ A teacher who is rigid and inflexible.

◆ A teacher who is boring and uncreative.

◆ A teacher who is disorganized.

◆ A teacher who can't be bothered to help you individually.

◆ A teacher who motivates through shame and criticism rather than praise and encouragement.

You and your parents should talk with your academic advisor about avoiding classes with "ADD-Toxic" teachers.

HIGH SCHOOL HASSLES

Accommodations for ADD in High School

There are laws requiring schools to accommodate your ADD so that you can be at your best in the classroom. One of the laws is called I.D.E.A., another is called Section 504 of the Rehabilitation Act. What you need to know is that you are protected by these laws, and have certain rights under them. One right is to have accommodations for your ADD in the classroom so that you can do your best work.

Some accommodations that have helped other high school students with ADD are:

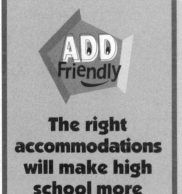

The right accommodations will make high school more ADD-Friendly.

1. Priority seating, near the front of the class and away from the classroom door—so that you can pay better attention and not be distracted by what's happening behind you or in the hall.

2. Extra time when taking tests.

3. A quiet, nondistracting place to take tests.

4. Customized scheduling of classes, so that you take your most difficult classes at the best times for you.

5. Special guidance during registration so you're assigned to the most "ADD-savvy" teachers at your school.

6. A second set of text books at home, so that you always have the books you need to do your homework.

7. A specially trained resource teacher, who can work with you to improve study skills, organization, and planning.

8. Having someone else complete "fill in the blank" exams for you if you are prone to make careless errors.

9. Be given alternative forms of examinations—for example, oral exams, or essay exams if short-answer and multiple-choice exams are particularly difficult for you.

Remember, getting accommodations for ADD is your <u>right.</u> Don't let anyone make you feel as if you're receiving an unfair advantage. Accommodations are meant to give you a chance to compete on more even terms with students who don't have ADD.

Talking to your Resource Teacher

If you are one of the lucky ones who has a resource teacher trained to help students with ADD, take advantage of the help! It may seem like an added hassle, but students who have an ADD resource teacher and meet with him/her regularly, do much better in school. What can a resource teacher do for you?

◆ They can talk to your teachers and explain the kinds of help you need.

◆ They can explain to your teachers that the problems you have are caused by ADD, not by laziness or irresponsibility.

◆ They can help you learn to be better organized, and keep up an assignment book.

◆ They can help you to stay focused and on-track.

◆ They can help you learn to problem-solve.

◆ They can help you practice explaining your needs so that you can become a better "self-advocate."

HIGH SCHOOL HASSLES

You should meet with your resource teacher at least once a week to review your papers, projects, and upcoming tests. Schedule a regular time to go so that you don't forget.

Taking tests

If you're like a lot of other students with ADD, taking tests is hard. Often students with ADD say:

"I really studied, but when I took the test I couldn't remember anything."

"I messed up because I didn't understand the directions."

"I didn't know I was supposed to know all that stuff for the exam."

"Essay exams are impossible for me. If they would just ask me, I could tell them the answer, but when I try to write it down, I freeze up."

"Multiple-choice tests are hard for me. Sometimes two answers seem correct, or, I can't tell the difference between them."

What can help to improve your test-taking ability?

◆ Take tests in a separate room. That way you will be less distracted and you can get up and walk around if you need to.

◆ Use extra time on tests—even if you say, "I always finish early." Having extra time gives you a chance to go back later and check for careless mistakes. You won't find them if you rush.

◆ Ask for exams to be administered in the way that's best for you. This includes oral exams if writing is hard for you, or essay exams, if short answers are difficult for you. You should also be given the chance to have someone fill in the "bubbles" on a multiple-choice exam if you tend to make lots of careless errors.

What if my teacher won't change a test for me?

These are "reasonable accommodations" under the law, but some teachers may not understand this. Sometimes you may need help to convince a teacher that you have a right to accommodations. Ask your tutor, resource teacher, or parent to help you negotiate with your teacher.

Learning How to Succeed in School

This section deals with

* Identifying your learning style

* Planning your day with day planners

* Planning projects/Completing projects

* Beating Procrastination

* Memorization tactics

* How to know when you "know" something

* When reading seems impossible

* Math/foreign languages

(continued on next page)

(continued from previous page)

✳ Computers and ADD

✳ Mental energy/Mental fatigue

✳ Dealing with distractions

✳ Working with a Tutor

Learning *how* to learn with ADD

Knowing how you learn best; learning how to study efficiently; how to stay organized; how to get your projects completed on time—all of these things are essential if you are going to become a successful student.

This section covers ways to become a more effective student. You may have already used some of these approaches, and others may be new to you. It can be helpful to work with a tutor who specializes in teaching high school students with ADD as you try to develop new habits and learning approaches.

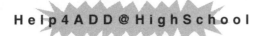
Identify Your Learning style

To learn best you need to know your learning style.

Our brains are not all alike. We each have a best-learning style. **If you study according to your learning style, you will learn information more quickly and retain it better.**

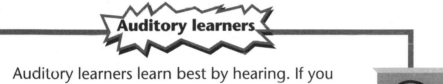

Auditory learners

Auditory learners learn best by hearing. If you are an auditory learner, you probably know how important it is for you to listen in class. Reading is visual and is sometimes harder for auditory learners.

Tips for auditory learners

◆ **Read aloud to yourself.**
This puts you in the auditory mode.

◆ **Talk about what you've read.**
This also reinforces the information in an auditory mode.

◆ **Speak aloud when you are memorizing**
names, terms, dates, etc.

◆ **Make up silly rhymes**
to remember information, like:

> *In fourteen hundred ninety-two*
> *Columbus sailed the ocean blue.*

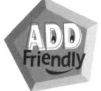

HOW TO SUCCEED IN SCHOOL

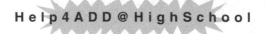
What to do in class:

If you are an auditory learner with ADD, you need to take full advantage of your listening strengths. Get all you can from class.

① Ask for **priority seating—front and center** in class. This means that you will have fewer distractions and can concentrate better on what you hear.

② Be sure your **most difficult classes** are during periods of the day **when you can listen best**—when your medication is at its peak, and when you are not sleepy in the morning, or too tired by the end of the day.

③ Ask **permission to tape classes** so that you can listen again to what the teacher said. This can be **especially important** if the teacher has a **review session** just before a big exam.

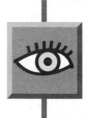

Visual learners

Visual learners learn best by seeing. If you are a visual learner, a class lecture may be "in one ear, out the other."

A good teacher for visual learners uses diagrams, charts, graphs, notes, and images to keep visual learners involved.

Tips for visual learners:

◆ **Be sure to take good notes.** Writing can help you stay focused and translates information from the auditory mode into the visual mode.

◆ If you have trouble taking notes, **get a copy of class notes.** The notes can come either from your teacher or from a student in class.

- **Use visual aids when you study:**
    Make charts and diagrams
    Draw silly pictures that can help you recall facts
    Use colored, felt-tipped pens and color-code
    your notes
    Ask people to *show you, not tell you,* when
    they explain something to you.

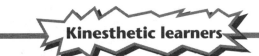

Kinesthetic learners

Kinesthetic learners. Kinesthetic learners learn best by doing. Learning in the classroom setting is hardest for kinesthetic learners.

Tips for kinesthetic learners

- **Use as many of your senses as you can** in the learning process. Use the auditory and visual modes together. In other words:
    See, say, read, and write.
- **Take as many classes as you can that have labs and workshops that provide "hands on" learning.**
- **Walk or pace while you read aloud.**
    Some students with ADD that are hyperactive, and especially ADD students who are kinesthetic learners, find they can stay focused and learn better if they stand or walk while reading aloud.
- **Jog while you listen to tapes.** Get permission to tape important classes—particularly review sessions before a big exam—and listen to the tape while you walk or jog.

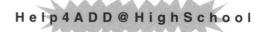

Plan

Planning your Day with Day planners

One public high school in the Washington, D.C., area has begun using the slogan, "If you plan to learn, you must learn to plan." They sell inexpensive day planners and require each student to use one.

This program has been so effective that some students who have transferred to other schools come back to purchase day planners!

> "If you plan to learn, you must learn to plan!"

What is a day planner? It is a book with a page for each day of the school year to record appointments, activities, and assignments.

A day planner can remind you of:

◆ Daily **homework** assignments in each class

◆ **Dates of quizzes and tests**

◆ **Due dates of papers and projects.**

A day planner can help you plan papers and projects:

◆ What are the steps of your project?

◆ What should you do first?

◆ When will you do it?

Learning to really use a day planner is probably one of the single most important changes you can make to become a better student.

Planning projects

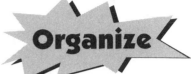
Organize

Learning to plan a project is a skill that you must develop. A "project" is a complicated, long-term assignment or task. All projects aren't class assignments.

You could have a project related to one of your extracurricular activities—such as working on the school newspaper or yearbook. Even planning a float for the homecoming parade is a complex project that needs to be planned!

You will need to learn how to plan a project.

Here are some suggestions:

1 Start with the "due date" of the project and plan backwards.

2 Break a big project into small steps.

3 Decide what is the best order to complete each small step.

4 Set a time and date for each of these small steps, and write them in your day planner.

5 If you need to work with someone else on some of the steps, plan this in advance. Make sure your parent, your lab partner, or whomever you need to work with is available at the planned time.

6 Make a big wall calendar for your project—mark the dates for each step of the project so that you can track your progress.

HOW TO SUCCEED IN SCHOOL

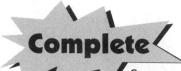

Complete

Completing projects

Some people with ADD have no problem in the "planning phase" of a project, but have lots of trouble finishing it. Here are some tips to help keep you on track:

1 Work as part of a team if possible. Other people working with you on the same project can help keep you on track.

2 If it is a solo project, work with a tutor or coach. This person can talk with you regularly about your progress, and can help you problem solve when you get off track.

3 When you feel overwhelmed . . .

Try "sneaking up" on your project. What do we mean by that? Don't make an ordeal of it! For example, don't set aside all weekend to work on it, and then feel so trapped that you can't work. Break it up. Work on your paper for half-an-hour before you leave for soccer practice. Grab 15 minutes before dinner to look up a reference on the Internet. Keep nibbling away at your project—don't try to swallow it whole!

4 Set deadlines for intermediate steps in the project. Make a commitment to these deadlines to your teacher or tutor.

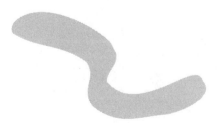

Beating Procrastination

Procrastination

Procrastination is often a big problem for students with ADD. Many teens with ADD get into the habit of beginning projects at the very last minute, and then stay up all night, or work all weekend to finish. They often miss deadlines, and receive lower grades on their paper or project as a result.

If you are a procrastinator, what can you do about it?

By understanding why you are procrastinating you'll have a better idea of how to overcome proscrastination..

◆ **Do you know where and how to begin?** You may procrastinate because you aren't sure how to get started. What should you do?

❶ Ask for help.

❷ Get clarification from your teacher.

❸ Work with your tutor.

◆ **Do you put it off because it feels too huge and over-whelming?**

❶ Try dividing your big paper or project into small, bite-sizes.

❷ Schedule short work periods at specific times.

◆ **Do you put off something because you just don't like doing it?**

❶ Try using the things you **want** to do as a reward for what you **need** to do.

❷ Use a phone call, a pizza, or a favorite TV show as a reward for having studied for an hour.

❸ Just be sure you don't give yourself the reward BEFORE you've earned it.

HOW TO SUCCEED IN SCHOOL

37

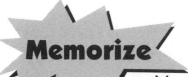

Memorization Tactics

Many students don't know how to learn and memorize information efficiently. They just read the information over and over, and then are surprised when they can't retrieve it for the test.

Here are some of the best tactics to memorize information for recall:

Chunk it!

Do you have a long list of facts to memorize? Chunk them into groups that belong together. Chunks can be made in any way that makes sense to you. A chunk could be:

All the bones in the leg
(if you are memorizing the bones of the body);

All the terms that begin with the letter "P;"

All the men who were President of the United States from 1900 to 1925.

Sing it!

Words put to music are easier to recall. Ever notice how easy it is for you to remember song lyrics?   The sequence of notes helps us to recall the sequence of words.

Rhyme it!

Rhymed facts are easy to recall. Song lyrics are easy to remember because they often rhyme. Make your rhyme a silly one—sometimes that's even easier to remember.

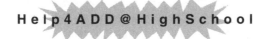

Acronym it!

Find a way to make up a word or abbreviation using the first letter of each word in the list—this is called an acronym.

Here are two acronyms that describe good ways to do paperwork:

The **KISS** method: Keep It Simple, Sweetheart!

The **OHIO** method: Only Handle It Once.

Associate it!

Associate a new fact with a familiar one. The more we can associate a fact with other things that we already know, the more likely we are to remember the new fact and be able to recall or retrieve it.

Visualize it!

Try to create a visual image that will help you to remember a fact. This approach is good for everyone, but is especially good for visual learners.

For instance, take the name of the author Thornton Wilder.

You might visualize a thorn for "Thornton;" maybe a thorn in a wild growth of bushes for "Wilder."

HOW TO SUCCEED IN SCHOOL

39

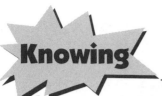

Knowing

How do you KNOW when you KNOW?

This may sound like a silly question, but many students aren't aware of different levels of knowing something.

1. Recognition level

> At the recognition level, when you see or hear something you "recognize" it.

Many students think that when they recognize something in the book, or in their notes, that they have studied enough. This level of learning is usually only adequate for responding to very easy multiple-choice questions such as:

The man who was President of the United States during the Civil War was:

      a) Mickey Mouse

      b) George Washington

      c) Walter Cronkite

      d) Abraham Lincoln

2. Retrieval level

> At the retrieval level, when you're asked a direct question you can "retrieve" that fact from your memory.

A retrieval level question would be:

Who was President of the United States during the Civil War?

A retrieval question gives you no hints—you have to retrieve the fact from memory.

3. Association level

> At the association level, you would be asked not only to retrieve a single fact, but to associate related facts as well.

An association level question might be:

Who was President of the United States during the Civil War, and what were the major events of his presidency?

40

Your teacher might expect you to mention:

    The Civil War

    Ulysses S. Grant

    The Gettysburg Address

    The Emancipation Proclamation

    Lincoln's assassination

4. Comprehension level

At this highest level, you understand and can explain the meaning and importance of the facts that you have learned and can retrieve.

A comprehension level question might be:

What were the social and economic forces existing in the northern and southern regions of the United States in the mid-nineteenth century which led to the outbreak of the Civil War?

You might be expected to discuss the differences between the South, which was a hierarchical, agrarian society, owned primarily by Anglo/Saxon families, who had immigrated to the colonies many generations ago, whose economy was highly dependent upon slave labor; and the northern U.S., which was much more heterogeneous, whose wealthy class had earned their money through commerce and industry rather than agriculture, and which was exploding with more recently arrived immigrants from many European countries.

As you can see, a student who "knows" enough about the Civil War to choose Abraham Lincoln's name in a multiple-choice question, might not be able to retrieve his name, associate it with other relevant facts, and comprehend the social and economic forces of the Civil War period.

Learning

So let's go back to our original questions:

How do you know when you "know" something?
What is the best way for you to learn it?

To really know something, you need to be able to:

❶ Pull facts from your memory bank

❷ Associate related facts

❸ Explain how they are related and why they are important.

Here are steps to take to REALLY know something:

Write down important facts from your text or notes

Read what you've written

Say what you've read

Think about what you've read

Explain in your own words what you've learned.

Sound like too much work? You'll be surprised how much more quickly your studying goes when you pay attention to your learning style and use it to study.

You'll also be amazed at how quickly the time goes when you are really involved in the learning process rather than bored and half-asleep on your bed as you try to study your "old" way.

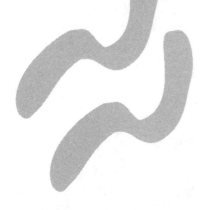

When reading seems impossible

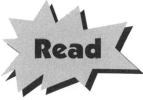
Read

Many students with ADD say that they "just can't read." No matter how hard they try, they find that when they start to read they feel sleepy or bored, and soon their mind is wandering while their eyes are scanning the page.

If reading is hard for you, here are some tips:

❶ Don't lie down while you read. You are tempting fate!

❷ Exercise frequently while reading and studying. One hyperactive student made a habit of 10 minutes on the treadmill every time he found himself feeling groggy and sleepy while reading.

❸ Read aloud—you'll feel more engaged, and you'll be using two of your senses—hearing and seeing.

❹ Use recorded books.

❺ Take notes while you read—one sentence for each paragraph of text.

❻ Underline—Underlining can help you pay better attention while you read, but is sometimes not as effective as note-taking. Why?

Because when you take notes, you are more actively involved by putting what you've read in your own words.

❼ Read when you're rested. Don't pick your "tired time" of day to read.

❽ Read frequently and in short bits—You'll maintain better concentration.

❾ Practice reading—it's a skill that improves with practice. If you are not a regular reader it will be harder and take more energy.

HOW TO SUCCEED IN SCHOOL

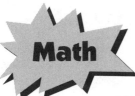

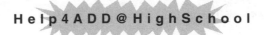

Many students with ADD experience difficulty with math courses. This may be due to a learning disability in the area of mathematics, or simply due to ADD patterns.

ADD patterns that get in the way of earning good math grades are:

❶ Careless errors

Take time to double-, and triple-check your answers.

❷ Poor handwriting, and crooked number columns lead to incorrect calculations.

Using large, square graph paper can help better organize problems as you are copying and solving them.

❸ Putting comprehension into practice.

Many ADD students find they understand a concept in class, but come home and can't do the homework. A tutor who can explain the concept, and sit with you while you put that understanding into action by working through assigned problems, can really help.

44

Foreign languages

Languages

Learning foreign languages can be hard for students with ADD. Why? Learning a foreign language **requires:**

◆ **attention to detail**

◆ **practice and discipline**

◆ **memory skills**

Many students with ADD experience difficulty with spelling, grammar, attention to detail, and memory when they are studying in English. These same problems are compounded when they try to study a foreign language.

Although most high schools require taking a foreign language, don't worry if you don't do well, or are unable to progress successfully through second and third years of a foreign language. Many colleges allow a foreign-language course substitution if you have proper documentation of foreign-language learning problems.

If you have difficulty with foreign languages, be sure to explore carefully language requirements of colleges to which you apply.

HOW TO SUCCEED IN SCHOOL

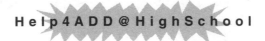

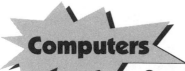

Computers

Computers are a real plus for high school students with ADD. Computers offer an easy solution to a few common ADD problems.

1 Many students with ADD have **poor handwriting.** Good penmanship requires patience, fine motor control, and attention to detail. By using a computer, your papers will be legible and much more appealing to your teachers.

2 **Spelling difficulties** also are common among students with ADD. With computer spell-check you can easily catch most spelling errors.

> **If you don't have good keyboarding skills, developing them must be a top priority.**

If you become a fast keyboarder, without needing to look at the keys as you write, your work will go very fast. There are excellent programs for developing keyboarding skills, but the challenge for most students with ADD is keeping at it in a disciplined way. It is often better to take a keyboarding class to make sure you get regular practice.

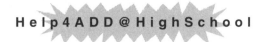

Mental energy/mental fatigue

Energy

Many students with ADD struggle with problems of mental fatigue.

Mental fatigue can be caused by:

1. Boredom

2. Prolonged mental effort

3. Working in an area of weakness

4. Working in your nonpreferred mode—such as reading if you are an auditory learner.

Ways to combat mental fatigue:

1. Stand up while listening.

2. Take a brief break from studying to walk around.

3. Change your focus—if you are studying for a history exam, it may help to do algebra homework for a while and then come back to your history studies.

4. Read or memorize while walking. This may sound funny, but hyperactive students are often able to study more effectively if they pace and read aloud while studying.

5. Study during your peak energy times.

ADD Friendly

HOW TO SUCCEED IN SCHOOL

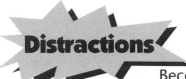
Distractions

Dealing with distractions

Becoming distracted is one of the biggest problems when a student with ADD tries to study.

Headphones or radio

Some students find that if they wear headphones and listen to music while they study that they're better able to concentrate because the music blocks out all other types of distractions. (Many parents, however, don't believe this and think that their teenager is just goofing off).

White noise

"White noise" is monotonous background noise such as the noise of a fan or air-conditioner. You can purchase small "white noise" machines that block out other sounds very effectively, but it's cheaper and easier to simply turn on a fan in your room.

Turn off temptations!

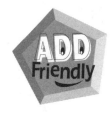

- ◆ Close your door
- ◆ Unplug the phone
- ◆ Turn off the TV
- ◆ Stay away from computer games!

Go to the library

If your room is still too distracting, even after trying all the approaches listed above, you may need to go to the library to study. But don't let the library become a place to socialize! This defeats your purpose in going there.

Working with a tutor

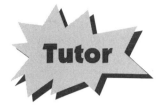

When working with a tutor, it's really important to find someone with whom you feel comfortable—someone who encourages you, not criticizes you.

A tutor can offer:

❶ Help with specific courses

❷ Help keep you on track and focused

❸ Help with writing problems such as:

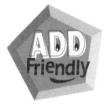

Mistakes in spelling and grammar

Accidentally omitting words and phrases

Difficulty organizing your ideas

❹ Help with Study Skills

You will need help in developing many of the study skills talked about in this section. Working with a tutor on a regular basis can make the process much easier.

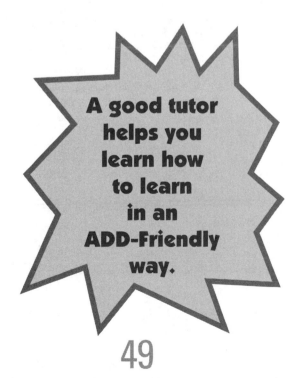

A good tutor helps you learn how to learn in an ADD-Friendly way.

HOW TO SUCCEED IN SCHOOL

Alternatives to Public High School

Private school?
G.E.D?
High school?

This section covers

* Private day school

* Boarding school

* Home schooling

* Earning your GED

* Therapeutic treatment programs

Private school

The last thing many high school students want to hear is that they should transfer to a private school. But if you've tried all the approaches we've talked about and you're still having lots of difficulty, then private school may be the next thing to consider. What might be better about a private school?

1. Smaller classes

◆ You're more likely to participate in small classes.

◆ It's more difficult to "hide" or sleep in class.

◆ You're more likely to ask questions when you don't understand something.

◆ There are fewer distractions.

2. More time with teachers

◆ Your teachers have more time to interact with you and to make sure you are "tuned in" during class.

◆ Your teachers will be able to give you more individual help outside of class.

3. More flexible programs

Public high schools are less flexible because they must meet the needs of many more students. Private schools can design a program for a particular type of student, and have much more flexibility to set up courses, schedules, and assignments in a custom-designed way.

> **Many students with ADD are more successful in small, private-school settings.**

Home Schooling

Some families choose the option of home schooling for their teenager with ADD. When a student is home-schooled, their studies are monitored by a parent.

Although they don't attend academic classes at high school, in some cases they may participate in clubs, sports, band, or other extracurricular activities at the local high school.

Home schooling is sometimes the best choice depending upon the student, his parent, and their ability to work together productively.

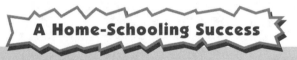

A Home-Schooling Success

Angie was a very bright, but highly distractible 8th grader who was struggling to keep up. Angie found middle school very confusing and distracting. She had difficulty keeping track of books, assignments, and changing from one classroom and teacher to another.

Beginning in 9th grade, Angie was home-schooled by her mother. Angie had always been a conscientious student who was close to her parents. She found when she studied at home that she could get her reading and assignments done in a few short hours each day. Angie's mother approached home schooling in a very organized way and this helped Angie to remain focused and organized.

Angie and her parents arranged for her to participate in a number of interesting volunteer projects in the community to fill her free time.

She lived near her high school and was able to participate in sports and extracurricular activities at the high school.

By her senior year, Angie chose to go to the public high school. She had only a few more requirements to fulfill and felt the pressures would not be too great. Home schooling had been very successful. As a senior, Angie felt ready to handle the stimulation and confusion of large classes.

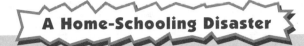

A Home-Schooling Disaster

Scott was a very gifted, but very undisciplined 9th grader, who seemed to have a knack for annoying most of his teachers. He never came to class prepared and often slept through class. Scott's mother felt defensive, angry, and worried, as she sat in teacher conference after teacher conference, where teachers vented their frustration over his continuing resistance to school requirements.

In complete frustration, Scott's mother decided to keep him home, and home school him in 10th grade.

Scott, unlike Angie, had very little internal motivation. Scott's mother, unlike Angie's mother, had little organizational ability herself, and did not have a cooperative working relationship with Scott. Scott began the school year by sleeping later and later in the morning.

When Scott arose around 10:30 or 11:00 a.m., he ate breakfast in front of the television. Then the nagging began, as his mother told him it was time to get dressed and come into the dining room where they had set up their "classroom." Scott resisted, saying that he was tired.

His friends from high school arrived home only three hours after Scott had crawled out of bed. Usually one or another of them called or dropped by.

Scott typically spent evenings in his room where he had access to his computer, his phone, and his television.

At the end of one year of home schooling, Scott's mother admitted defeat and informed Scott that he would be enrolled in a private school with small classes for the coming fall term. Low motivaton and lack of structure had made Scott's home schooling a failure.

Home schooling can be an excellent option for the right student with ADD. It can relieve many of the distractions and pressures of a large, public high school. However, before you or your family consider a home-schooling option, you need to honestly consider whether you are more like Angie or more like Scott!

Quitting high school and earning your GED

Some students with ADD, for many different reasons, can't seem to find an option in high school that works for them. If you have tried treatment, tutoring, psychotherapy, medication, and private school, and are still getting failing grades, then you may want to consider quitting school and taking the exam to earn your General Equivalency Diploma (GED). This is a high school equivalency degree, which can allow you to enter your local community college.

What are the pluses of quitting school and taking the GED?

◆ Your high school frustrations are over.

◆ You can quit the constant battling with your worried, frustrated parents over homework and grades.

◆ You can spend time and energy focusing on your future.

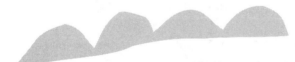

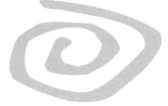

What's the down side of quitting school?

◆ You may feel very isolated.

◆ Your college choices are very limited.

◆ Your job prospects will be very limited and low paying.

◆ You may feel lost as you try to decide where to go and what to do next.

Don't make the choice to quit school unless all of your other options have failed.

Therapeutic treatment programs

There are a few schools especially designed for teens struggling with overwhelming problems such as: drug or alcohol abuse; depression and/or anxiety; and learning and attentional problems. These are usually called "treatment programs" rather than boarding schools. Most teens with ADD never need this kind of intensive program. But for some students, these therapeutic schools have really helped them turn their lives around. The schools usually have very small classes, very flexible teaching programs, and provide psychotherapy, group therapy, and other forms of treatment to help with coexisting conditions such as addiction, anxiety, and depression.

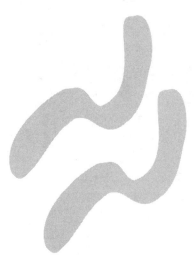

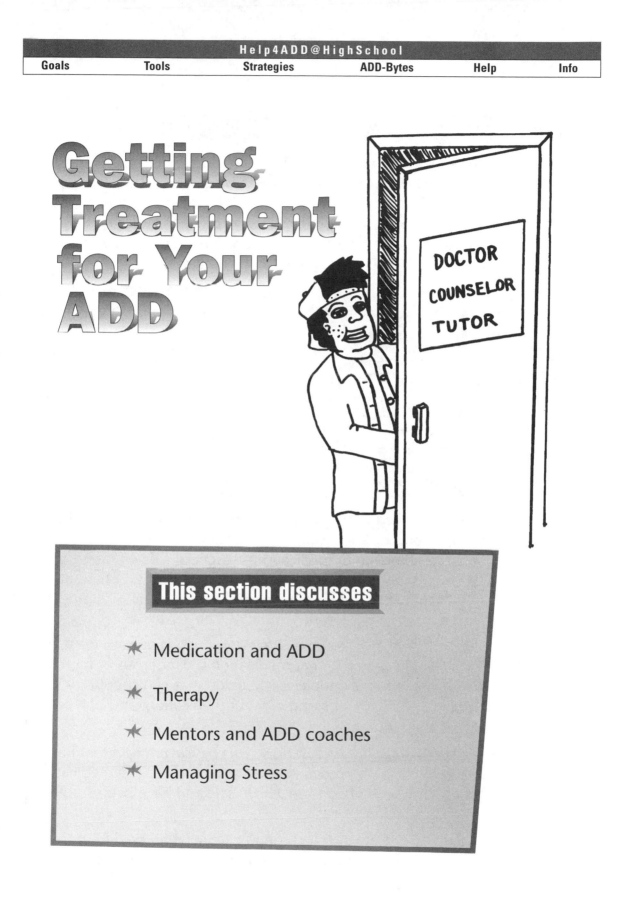

Getting Treatment for Your ADD

DOCTOR
COUNSELOR
TUTOR

This section discusses

* Medication and ADD

* Therapy

* Mentors and ADD coaches

* Managing Stress

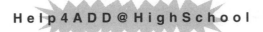
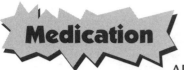
Medication

Medication and ADD

ADD is a neurobiochemical disorder. This means that the chemistry and structure of your brain is different when you have ADD. Medication increases the availability of important neurochemicals in your brain so that you can concentrate, plan, organize, and remember better. You will need to see a doctor specializing in ADD who can prescribe medication.

The most appropriate medications for ADD are stimulants which turn on those areas of the brain that aren't working as well as they should.

There are several types of stimulants.

The most common stimulants prescribed for treating ADD are:

◆ **Ritalin**

◆ **Dexedrine**

◆ **Adderol**

You may need to try more than one before you find the medication that works best for you. Many times a doctor will prescribe a combination of medications—especially if you have problems with sleep; with feeling tense or anxious; or have problems with depression. Some antidepressants also help ADD symptoms.

You may hear from friends or even from your parents, that medication is dangerous or harmful. Some people may tell you that you should try hard to get along without medication, and only take it as a last resort.

It is NOT true that stimulant medication is dangerous.

ADD is a *real physical problem* that has a proven effective treatment. The medications prescribed for ADD are safe and have been studied for a long time.

Taking medication can help you benefit more from tutoring, and can help you take charge of your ADD.

Medication side effects

Everyone responds differently to medication. If you experience headaches, stomachaches, or jittery feelings while on a stimulant medication, you may need to adjust your dose or try a different medication. Or, you may need to take a second medication in combination with the stimulant. For example, people who are prone to feeling tense and anxious often need to take an antide-pressant medication with a stimulant medication.

Most people with ADD have a positive reaction to medication and can really benefit from taking it every day.

How do you know if medication is helping?

Sometimes you may not see yourself very accurately. It can be hard to step back and look at yourself objectively. If you're not sure whether your medication is helping, ask your parents and your teachers if they have noticed improvements in your ADD patterns.

What changes should you look for when you take medication?

- Better able to listen in class

- Better able to keep your mind on what you're reading

- More organized in going through your day

- Feel less tense and frazzled

- Lose your temper less often

- Don't feel mentally wiped out at the end of the school day

GETTING TREATMENT

Sharing medication with friends

Because stimulants ARE so helpful, your friends may ask you to share some with them if they need to "pull an all nighter." **Don't share your meds!**

These have been specially prescribed for you because you have a real need for them. If your doctor thinks you are misusing or abusing your stimulant medication, he'll quit prescribing it, and then you're the one who will lose out.

Besides, it's illegal to distribute (share) prescription medication.

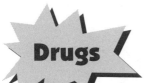

Drugs

Doing Drugs—Self-medication

It's not logical, but lots of teens with ADD who say they don't want to take medicine, are actually trying to treat their ADD through "self-medication" in ways that are bad for them.

Nicotine and caffeine

Many teens with ADD are attracted to cigarettes and colas, coffee, or tea because of the stimulants in them. Cigarettes contain nicotine, a powerful stimulant; caffeine-rich soft drinks and coffee contain caffeine, another stimulant. The problem is that these stimulants are much harder on your body in large doses, not to mention the risk of lung cancer and emphysema from smoking.

Marijuana and alcohol

When you feel tense, frantic, overwhelmed or bummed out, and don't know that the problem is untreated ADD, you may be drawn to marijuana or alcohol because they'll make you feel temporarily relaxed or calm. The problem with alcohol or marijuana is:

◆ They are addictive.

◆ They may make you feel temporarily better, but overall you will function worse if you abuse alcohol or marijuana.

◆ Marijuana is illegal, so you're risking a lot to feel temporarily better.

Cocaine

Some teens with ADD who have experimented with cocaine report an interesting thing. While their friends get high on cocaine, they say that they feel much more focused and able to function.

So why shouldn't you take cocaine if it helps you to function better?

Because it's highly addictive and illegal. Taking cocaine can also kill you, especially if you are taking other stimulants!

Taking prescription stimulant medication according to your doctor's orders, is a safe, effective, legal, and non-addictive way to achieve the same goal.

Experimenting with other drugs

We're not going to make the "just say no" speech you've heard a thousand times. But what you should know is:

Teens with ADD are often attracted to drugs because they are looking for ways to feel better. It's a much better choice to take medication that has been carefully prescribed for you than to fool around with harmful and/or illegal drugs.

Your brain chemistry is already imbalanced—why take drugs that will just mess it up more? You're trying to straighten out your brain functioning so that things will go better. So, do yourself a favor, and don't mess your brain up with drugs.

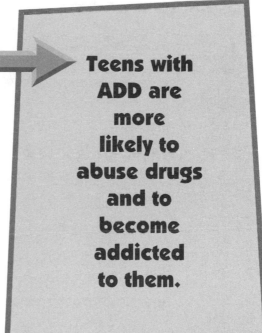

Teens with ADD are more likely to abuse drugs and to become addicted to them.

GETTING TREATMENT

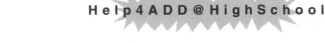

Coaches

Mentors and coaches

Therapists aren't the only ones who can help you with ADD in high school. There are other professionals who may be helpful in different ways.

> **A mentor** is someone older, whom you can look up to and can give you good advice, and be a role model for you. This could be a teacher whom you really like and who understands you. It might be an adult in the community—your music teacher, your athletic coach—someone who can help you recognize the best in youself and teach you how to build a future.

> **An ADD coach** is someone who works with you to help keep you on track as you work toward goals.

Coaching is one of the best ways to deal with your ADD. A coach can help you:

- ◆ Get organized
- ◆ Set goals
- ◆ Stay focused
- ◆ Solve problems
- ◆ Finish papers and projects
- ◆ Learn how to manage your time.

A coach provides external structure and support, and teaches how to develop your own internal structure. You might meet weekly or more often with an ADD coach. Some coaches also make quick, phone check-in calls between your appointments to help keep you on track.

Therapy

Therapy for ADD shouldn't be just talking about feelings, although that's important. It should also focus on practical ways to help you feel better and function better.

ADD therapy should:

① Help you UNDERSTAND ADD and exactly how it affects YOU.

② Help you RECOGNIZE YOUR STRENGTHS, not just focus on problems.

③ Help you SOLVE PROBLEMS, not just talk about them.

④ Teach you tools that help you "GET YOUR ACT TOGETHER."

⑤ Help you make good decisions about WHAT TO DO AFTER HIGH SCHOOL.

⑥ Help improve communication and REDUCE HASSLES BETWEEN YOU AND YOUR PARENTS.

Let's look at some of the most common problems that teens with ADD face, and how therapy helps to solve them.

GETTING TREATMENT

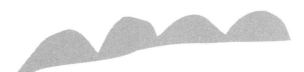

Anxiety and Depression

When your life just feels overwhelming

Many teens with ADD suffer from anxiety and depression which needs to be treated along with their ADD.

▶ **Anxiety—you may have anxiety if you answer "yes" to:**

1 I worry all the time about little things.

2 Sometimes I worry so much that I have trouble going to sleep.

3 I almost never feel relaxed.

4 I feel very self-conscious and am easily embarrassed.

5 Sometimes I feel so overwhelmed by problems at school that I pretend to be sick so that I can stay home.

6 I often feel nervous and jittery.

▶ **Depression—you may be depressed if you answer "yes" to:**

1 The future looks really bad to me.

2 I rarely feel excited or interested in things.

3 I have trouble sleeping, or sleep "all the time."

4 My eating has changed a lot (either overeating or no appetite).

5 I feel tired and irritable much of the time.

6 I feel little energy to "get going" on things I need to do.

When to seek treatment for anxiety or depression

If you feel that you would answer "yes" to many of the statements above, talk to your doctor or therapist. You don't have to keep on feeling badly. There are many new medications that are safe and have very few side effects. They can help you feel good again. But medication alone is not enough. It's important to talk to a therapist regularly if you are anxious or depressed.

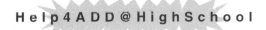

The effect of years of criticism for ADD behaviors ➤ **Blaming Yourself**

Do you blame yourself, or do your parents and teachers blame you for:

◆ Being "lazy"

◆ Not trying hard enough

◆ Lacking self-discipline

◆ Being a "slob."

If you feel discouraged about yourself, there are many things you can do to feel better. Your counselor or therapist can support you in making these changes.

GETTING TREATMENT

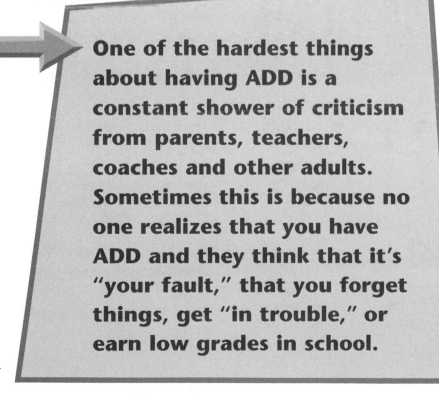

One of the hardest things about having ADD is a constant shower of criticism from parents, teachers, coaches and other adults. Sometimes this is because no one realizes that you have ADD and they think that it's "your fault," that you forget things, get "in trouble," or earn low grades in school.

Improving Self-Esteem

Therapy can be an important step toward feeling better about yourself. A therapist can help you quit blaming yourself, and help you take steps to emphasize your positive side.

There are many things that can help you feel good about yourself.

Here are a few of them:

❶ **Look for a support group of other teens who have ADD**—at school or in your local CHADD group. Talking with other teens who have struggled with the same sorts of problems can help you feel less alone.

> **What can you do to feel better about yourself?**

❷ **Get in touch with your strengths and your gifts.**
School is often not the best place for you to show off your talents if you have ADD. You've spent most of your life in school and haven't had a chance to test your abilities in other environments. Lots of people who are tremendous successes in their lives were not happy during their school years, and were not "good students." Get involved in volunteer activities, part-time work, or extracurricular activities. You'll be surprised at the interests and talents you'll discover.

❸ **Learn more about ADD by reading books like this.** The more you understand about yourself and ADD, the less likely you'll see yourself as unsuccessful. ADD is a difference, but it doesn't have to be a disability—you just need to put yourself in the right spot to take advantage of your strengths, talents, and energy.

❹ **Hang out with people who like and appreciate you.** Look for teachers, counselors, and friends who recognize the things you are really good at, and who don't dwell on your problems.

Losing Your temper

Some teens with ADD have a problem with losing their tempers very easily. Here are some of the reasons why:

Defending yourself from hurt feelings

Having an angry explosion will temporarily get people to leave you alone when your feelings have been hurt. The problem is that you end up feeling worse, and you're even less likely to get positive responses from others after an explosion.

Exploding due to a "chemical imbalance"

Sometimes teens with ADD have a kind of chemical imbalance in their brains that makes them get very, very frustrated over little things. Some teens report they feel enormous pressure and tension and can feel an explosion coming on, but can't seem to stop themselves even when they try.

Anger reactions due to tension and frustration

When you've had a bad day, you may explode at the slightest thing. Your angry reaction may seem very justified at the time, but chances are that you'll feel badly, even a little ashamed after it's over.

Acting angry instead of acting scared or worried

Sometimes it feels safer to get angry than to feel vulnerable. Often, boys are taught not to admit feeling scared or worried. When they do feel scared, the emotion they show the world is anger. Girls sometimes hide their feelings with anger also.

OK, we've listed some reasons why you may have an anger problem, but what can you do about it?

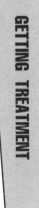

GETTING TREATMENT

Anger Management

Things to do when your anger causes problems.

1 Talk to your counselor to figure out what feelings and patterns are causing angry outbursts. Once you understand more, you and your counselor can start problem-solving.

Your counselor or therapist can help you think about your angry outbursts and possible solutions. He or she can help explore the patterns that lead to your explosions and figure out ways to reduce or eliminate them.

2 Stimulant medication for ADD often helps to control temper reactions. It helps you to stop and think about what you're doing before you do it. Most of the time, if you took a second to stop and think you'd still feel angry, but you might not react the same way.

3 Get away from the situation which is making you feel so frustrated. Take a break from your math homework if you're feeling stuck and frustrated. Get away from your little brother if he's bugging you and you're feeling stressed out.

4 Apologize when you've hurt someone's feelings. An apology doesn't make what you did OK, but at least you've let the other person know you're sorry, and you're trying to learn better ways to cope with your anger.

5 Take a break from the debate. If you're asking to borrow the car and your parents say "no," you may feel like yelling at them. It may help to leave the situation until you're calmer. You're much more likely to convince your parents to see it your way if you can come back and talk about it calmly.

68

Strategies for Problem ADD Patterns

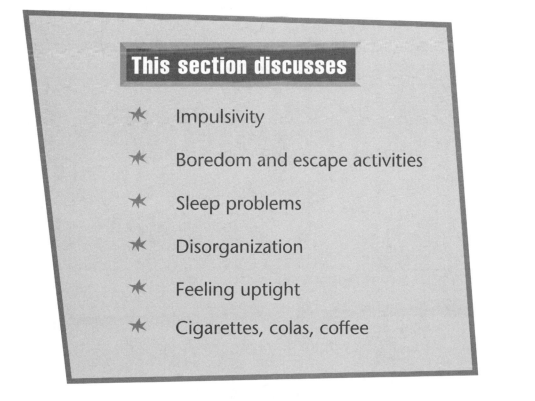

This section discusses

* Impulsivity

* Boredom and escape activities

* Sleep problems

* Disorganization

* Feeling uptight

* Cigarettes, colas, coffee

Impulsivity

Impulsivity

Impulsivity

Many teenagers have a tendency to do things on impulse. If you are a teen with ADD, you are even more likely to be impulsive. Why are impulsive actions a problem? They aren't always "bad," but doing things impulsively means that you haven't stopped to think about what might happen. What are some typical teen ADD impulses?

Quitting something when you're frustrated

Many teens with ADD get to a certain point and give up because they're discouraged or frustrated.

Often you may quit something that you really care about and this hurts you. You may quit a job on impulse because you've overslept once again and don't want to face the boss. You may quit a sports team because the coach yelled at you, or quit a project because it seemed too hard.

What to do besides impulsively quitting:

1. Give yourself some time to cool off before you make a decision.

2. Talk to someone you trust about the problem. They might help you see the problem in a different way.

3. Get some help if a project seems too difficult.

4. Reward yourself for sticking with a difficult task. If you don't stick with it, you'll never have the satisfaction of learning how to get through the rough spots and coming out a winner on the other side.

Impulsively "getting in trouble"

Many teens with ADD get into trouble with their parents, with the school, even with the police, not because they are "bad" and don't care about the rules, but because they did something impulsively such as:

- ◆ drink and drive
- ◆ paint graffiti on the school walls
- ◆ sneak out with a friend after curfew
- ◆ experiment with drugs offered to you at a party
- ◆ have unprotected sex.

You don't have to be perfect—all teenagers like to spread their wings, stretch the rules a little, have some fun. But when your impulsive act lands you in jail, gets you pregnant, or abusing drugs, then you will pay for your impulsivity for a long time.

Don't inflict disastrous consequences on yourself for a moment's impulse. Think ahead about what you'll do when your friends encourage you to do something you'll regret.

❶ Make sure there is a designated driver if you are going to a party and expect to drink.

❷ Get permission to spend the night so that you don't have to drink and drive.

❸ Always carry a condom if you are sexually active.

❹ Look for "safe" thrills—that won't risk the lives of other people and won't get you arrested, like rock climbing, mountain biking, or skiing.

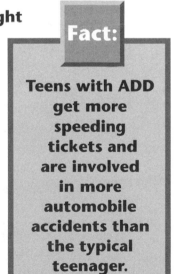

Fact:

Teens with ADD get more speeding tickets and are involved in more automobile accidents than the typical teenager.

STRATEGIES FOR ADD PATTERNS

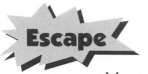

Boredom and Escape Activities

Many teens with ADD complain of boredom. They have trouble thinking of interesting things to do and end up spending lots of time as a *couch potato; watching television, or playing computer games.* More and more teens with ADD are becoming almost *addicted to on-line interaction with other teens.*

What's the problem with these kinds of activities? Nothing if they are done in moderation, but many teens with ADD get "hooked" on TV, games, or on-line chats.

Why are escape activities so appealing?
- ◆ They are easy—no sweat
- ◆ They are always there
- ◆ You don't have to plan anything
- ◆ You don't have to challenge your brain
- ◆ You don't have to organize anything

Escape activities are just "there" waiting for you

"So what's wrong with that?," you ask. The problem is not with what you're doing, but with all the things you are *not* doing—like exercise, sports, hobbies, or skill-building activities. Teenage and young adult years should be years of excitement, of trying new things—of learning what you're good at and what you care about. If you spend high school plugged into America OnLine (AOL), watching reruns on TV, and playing Super Mario on Nintendo, you've kept yourself from all the excitement and learning available out in the "real world."

School sports can help you learn self-discipline, and how to learn to cooperate and coordinate with others. Hobbies you develop in high school may turn into a career option later. Participating in school projects and activities can help you grow and develop in ways you may never imagine.

Instead of escaping into dead-end activities, why not explore, excite, and challenge yourself to find what you're good at while doing new things?

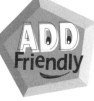

Sleep Problems

High school schedules are very badly designed for teenagers. Most teenagers like to stay up late and sleep late, but have to get up at the crack of dawn to be at school on time. That means that lots of teens never really get enough sleep during the week.

Many people with ADD are natural "night owls." No matter how tired they may feel during the day, they find that they "wake up" in the evening and don't feel sleepy at bedtime.

What are some things to do to help yourself get to sleep?

1 **Get into a regular routine.** Our bodies respond to routines. If you always turn the light out around 11 p.m., then your body will be trained to feel sleepy around 11 p.m.

2 **Don't do things in the evening that are going to get you wound up**—like talk on the phone until the minute before you're supposed to go to sleep; or have a fight with your Mom over whether you have to come home and mow the lawn after school tomorrow.

3 **Do something relaxing during the hour before bed.** Take a warm shower, get in bed and read quietly.

4 **Play quiet, relaxing music if you are distracted by sounds in the house and can't sleep.**

5 **If you just can't get to sleep, read a book.** Don't watch TV, don't use the computer, don't start playing Nintendo. Read homework assignments. Reading often puts people to sleep, and if it doesn't, at least you're getting some homework done!

6 **Get regular exercise.** If you are hyperactive, or even just restless and fidgety, you need exercise every day to really feel tired at night. But don't exercise just before bedtime! That tends to wake people up.

Feeling chronically tired during the week will make your ADD symptoms worse. Getting enough sleep is a very important way to learn to reduce your ADD symptoms.

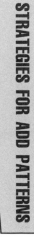

STRATEGIES FOR ADD PATTERNS

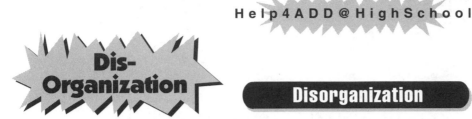

Disorganization

Disorganization is one of the biggest challenges of having ADD. When you are a kid, your parents and teachers do most of the organizing for you, but as you go through high school, you are expected to do more and more of it for yourself.

Getting organized isn't about being hassled by your mom to clean up your room, or getting hassled by your dad to remember to take out the trash or mow the lawn.

> **Getting organized is about learning to accomplish things that *you* want to accomplish.**

Lots of teenagers spend so much energy resisting the adults in their lives telling them to get their acts together, that they never understand the need to get their acts together for themselves.

Remember:
Being disorganized isn't just a hassle for your parents! Disorganization gets in YOUR way big time.

When you set goals for yourself, being organized is the way to meet them.

Getting organized can be divided into two main categories:

❶ **Organizing your time**—
  ◆ what you do with your time
  ◆ when you do it

❷ **Organizing your things**—
having your papers, books, and belongings in places where you can find them when you need them.

There are many techniques for helping people with ADD get organized. For teens with ADD, the best approach is to work with a coach or tutor on developing organizational skills.

74

Relaxation

Feeling uptight

There are important "therapeutic" exercises you can learn to lower your stress level and relax. These are very important tools for managing the negative side of ADD.

Some relaxation exercises are:

1 Controlled deep breathing

2 Progressive muscle relaxation

3 Visualization

4 Meditation

Your therapist can teach you some of these techniques. They are excellent tools to develop, and can help you better control your emotions. Relaxation techniques can help you get to sleep at night and help you feel less anxious in upsetting situations.

Cigarettes, Colas, Coffee

Many teens with ADD are attracted to cigarettes, colas, and coffee because the caffeine and nicotine help them feel more alert and focused. We don't need to make the "smoking's bad for you" speech here—you already know that. But you may not know that if you have ADD, you are more likely to become addicted to cigarettes, and use colas and coffee almost like a medication. Medications prescribed for your ADD by a doctor are much safer and more effective. If you already smoke, you may find that it's easier to quit smoking if you get medication for your ADD. (More about this on p. 60).

STRATEGIES FOR ADD PATTERNS

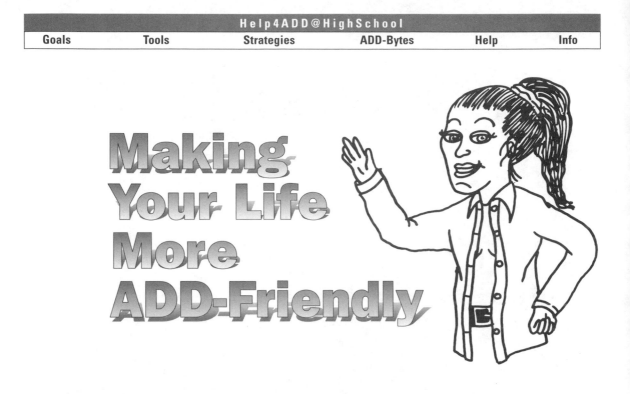

Making Your Life More ADD-Friendly

This section discusses

* Creating an ADD-Friendly life

* Taking good physical care of yourself

* Paying attention to your stress level

* Emphasizing the positive;
  downplaying the negative

* Do what you love

* Problem-solving—
  not problem-avoiding

* Confidence-building activities

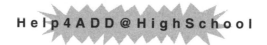
Creating an ADD-Friendly Life

We've talked about "ADD-Friendly" throughout this book. This idea is important because the most effective way to take charge of your ADD is to create a life that's designed to reduce negative ADD symptoms.

There are many things you can do in high school to make your life more ADD-Friendly. And when you get out of high school, there are more ways to create an ADD-Friendly life for yourself because you'll have more choices.

Right now, you don't have a lot of control over how you spend your day during school, although there are several things you CAN do, which we talked about in the section called "High School Hassles." Now, in this section, we're going to focus on things you can do for yourself that are separate from school issues.

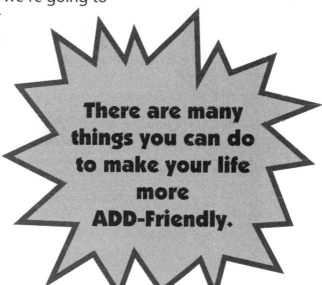

There are many things you can do to make your life more ADD-Friendly.

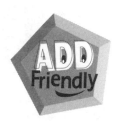

Health

Taking good physical care of yourself

You might ask—what does our physical state have to do with ADD? ADD symptoms are worse when we are tired, hungry, suffering from allergies, sick with a cold or with something more serious.

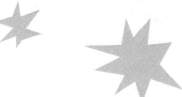

What can you do to reduce ADD symptoms?

- ◆ Get enough sleep
- ◆ Eat a healthy diet
- ◆ Eat often enough to avoid feeling "ravenous"
- ◆ Exercise every day
- ◆ Avoid too much caffeine
- ◆ Don't smoke cigarettes
- ◆ Don't abuse alcohol or drugs
- ◆ Take vitamins
- ◆ Go to the doctor before you get really sick

Stress

Pay attention to your stress level

Stress affects teens with ADD even more than it affects other teens. Stress is created by worry, tension, problems at home, conflicts with friends, deadlines, grade pressure, and college applications to name a few. ADD patterns such as chronic lateness, disorganization, and procrastination also create stress.

What can you do to manage your stress level?

1 Don't live in a "crisis mode"—i.e., not doing anything about your problems until they are really serious.

2 Work hard at being early. Running late all the time, rushing to get to work or to class creates tremendous stress.

3 Get help to reduce conflicts with people in your life— frequent fights and arguments are very stress-increasing.

4 Learn and practice relaxation techniques such as:
      Listening to relaxing music;
      Controlled deep breathing; and
      Yoga.

5 Identify stress reducers and use them!
      Take a walk;
      Take a hot bath;
      Give yourself a quiet "time out."

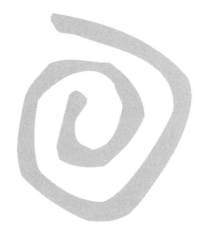

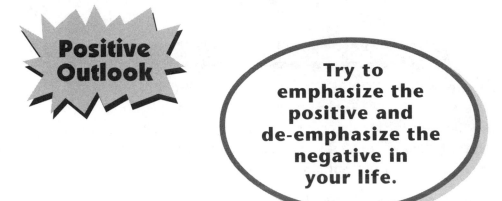

Positive Outlook

Try to emphasize the positive and de-emphasize the negative in your life.

❶ Look for positive interactions with people—people you enjoy; people who appreciate you and recognize what is best about you.

❷ Look for positive experiences—school may seem hard, boring, or endlessly frustrating at times, but you can offset these feelings by engaging in positive activities after school and on weekends. Choose activities that remind you that there are things in life that you are good at and enjoy.

❸ Even if school "isn't for you," lots of choices are just around the corner! Don't lose sight of them.

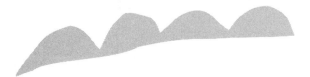

Do what you love

Interest

One of the best ways to reduce ADD symptoms is to do something you love. If you are really interested in an activity and enjoy it, you will find that you are much more focused and effective. Keep this in mind after high school. Look for a career path related to something you really enjoy and care about, and your chances for success will be MUCH greater.

- Don't let your parents or teachers convince you that you have to settle for doing something you dislike.

- Dare to dream.

  But be a realistic dreamer—think about ways to reach your dream.

- Think about unique or different ways to get where you want to go.

  School isn't always the answer!

- Doing something you really like and are interested in will let you positively direct your energy and creativity.

- Become partners with other people if you don't have all the skills or abilities to reach your goal.

- Work with a coach or counselor to keep you on the right track in pursuing your goals.

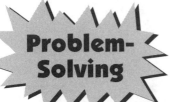

Problem-Solving

Problem-solving

Work on becoming a "problem-solver" rather than a "problem-avoider." This is something good to work on with a counselor who is an ADD specialist. Think of this approach as a challenge—looking for creative solutions when you encounter a problem instead of just feeling angry and frustrated.

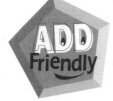

Steps in problem-solving:

❶ Define the problem in concrete terms.

❷ Examine why you think the problem exists.

❸ Brainstorm possible solutions.

❹ Choose the solution you think has the best chance to succeed.

❺ Try the solution.

❻ Evaluate whether this approach was successful.

❼ If not, think about why not.

❽ Try another solution.

❾ Keep up the good work—you'll get there!!

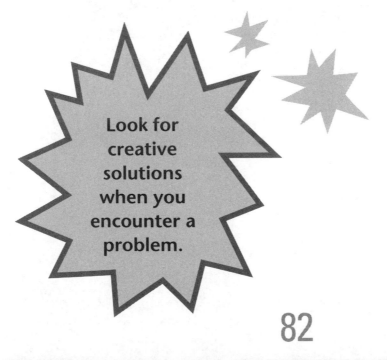

Look for creative solutions when you encounter a problem.

Confidence-Building Activities

Confidence

Look for activities that can be confidence builders for you. Many teens with ADD don't experience school as a confidence builder. Even if they are bright, many teens with ADD feel less successful in school than their peers.

What kinds of things can build your confidence? It's not the same for everyone, but some of the things that have helped other high school students feel more confident are:

- ◆ Sports

- ◆ Good friends

- ◆ Hobbies at which they can excel

- ◆ Summer or after-school jobs

- ◆ Outward Bound types of activities

- ◆ Singing, acting, or playing a musical instrument

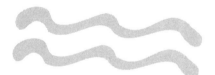

Developing confidence will help you tackle ADD challenges.

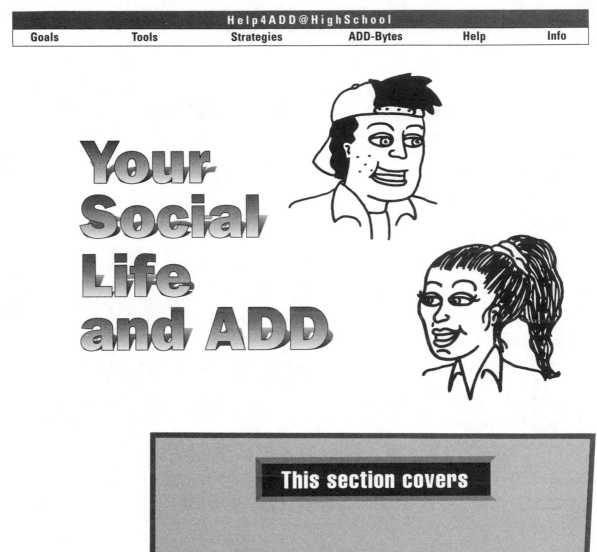

Your Social Life and ADD

This section covers

* Friends

* Dating

* Hiding behind roles

* When your social life becomes "everything" to you

Friends

Having good friends is really important during high school years, but it's crucial to find friends who are good for you.

Figuring out who is "good for you"

Some teens with ADD feel discouraged about themselves. They may feel they have few talents or accomplishments. As a result, many may be drawn to friends who have similar or even bigger problems.

There's nothing wrong with looking for people who understand you and are sympathetic. In fact, this is a good thing to do. But sometimes, friends who feel badly about themselves don't want you to improve your life because then they'll feel left behind.

Don't stay with friends who want you to stay "down" with them.

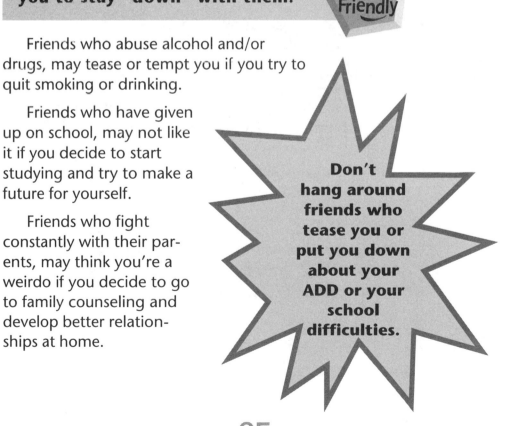

Friends who abuse alcohol and/or drugs, may tease or tempt you if you try to quit smoking or drinking.

Friends who have given up on school, may not like it if you decide to start studying and try to make a future for yourself.

Friends who fight constantly with their parents, may think you're a weirdo if you decide to go to family counseling and develop better relationships at home.

Don't hang around friends who tease you or put you down about your ADD or your school difficulties.

YOUR SOCIAL LIFE AND ADD

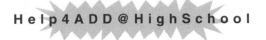
Changing yourself, changing your friends

One of the things you may notice when you start taking charge of your ADD, and feeling better about yourself, and making good decisions for your future, is that you don't fit in with the same friends anymore.

It's hard to change friends overnight , and it usually happens gradually. You may decide to try out for sports because you feel more confident, or try out for the school play. Gradually you'll find that you're hanging out with a different group of friends.

Although change is hard, this kind of change is really good. We usually feel most comfortable with friends when we have a lot in common with them. As you begin to feel more in charge of yourself, and more positive about your future, chances are that you will choose friends who feel the same —friends who feel good about themselves and good about you.

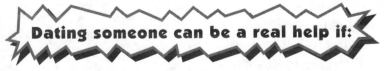

Does dating help you function better?

Some teens with ADD put most of their energy into their girl-friends or boyfriends because that's the main thing in their lives that makes them feel good.

You need to ask yourself whether dating helps you or is hurting you.

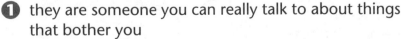

1 they are someone you can really talk to about things that bother you

2 they help you to think about problems and find better solutions

3 they are good at calming you down and getting you back on track.

4. they encourage you to get things done that you need to do—like study for tests, finish your papers, and do things you need to at home.

5. they understand how your ADD affects you and are patient when you "lose it" sometimes.

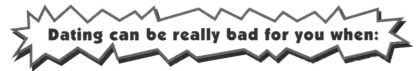

Dating can be really bad for you when:

1. your boyfriend or girlfriend wants all of your time and attention and makes it even harder for you to study and do other things you need to do.

2. you have so many fights and disagreements with your boyfriend or girlfriend that it keeps you upset.

3. you stay up too late at night talking on the phone with them.

4. when they don't understand your ADD and maybe don't even believe in ADD.

5. when they pick on you, criticize you, and generally make you feel less confident than you did before.

6. when they are having so many problems that they want you to pay attention to their needs and not to your own.

7. when they are involved in drug or alcohol abuse and encourage you to join them.

8. when they aren't working toward a positive future, and don't encourage you to take steps to have a positive future for yourself.

YOUR SOCIAL LIFE AND ADD

Basically you need to ask yourself, "is this person pulling me up, or pulling me down?" Your ADD is a big enough challenge. The last thing you need is someone in your life who makes it even harder to function. If you are lucky enough to find someone who cares, understands, and is supportive, then he or she can be a big help to you in learning how to take charge of your ADD.

Hiding Behind a Role

Some teens with ADD feel bad because they have poor grades or because they don't excel in sports. This may be true, not for lack of talent, but because it's hard for you to stick to anything long enough to become proficient at it. To make up for this, some teens with ADD take on a role—like "class clown," "life of the party," or guy or girl with a "bad attitude." By entertaining others, drinking and partying, showing off, breaking rules, or defying authority, these teens try to gain acceptance from their peers. The problem is that these roles are really a way to hide bad feelings about yourself.

It works a lot better to get treatment for your ADD, through counseling, coaching, and medication so that you can get the "good" attention you're afraid you'll never have. Once you take charge of your ADD, you won't need to hide behind a role. You'll be proud of just being yourself.

When Your Social Life Is Your Whole Life

A social life is crucial for most teens. And that's good. This is a time in life to become more independent from your parents and to rely more on peers for support, understanding, and interaction. The problem comes when your social life takes over, and you don't devote enough time to studying, learning, and developing skills. Students with ADD, who may not feel they can do well in school, may be tempted to get all of their positive strokes from friends.

Don't let your social life take over your whole life! Look for friends who will support and encourage you to earn better grades. Get experience in volunteer work and part-time jobs. Look for friends who will encourage you to build a positive future.

Girls With ADD

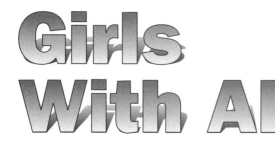 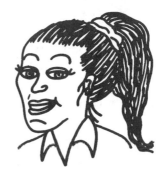

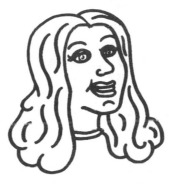

This section deals with

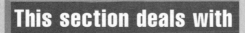

* Emotions

* ADD Patterns in Girls

* Social Issues

* Conflicts with Parents

* Feeling Ashamed

* Strengths for Girls with ADD

> If you are a teenage girl with ADD, you will need to cope with a few issues that are different from guys with ADD.

Emotions

Girls, in general, tend to be more emotionally expressive than guys. For girls with ADD, this is even more true. Girls with ADD typically have very intense emotional reactions—happiness, excitement, embarrassment, anger, self-consciousness, sadness and anxiety. One way to think of this is that **guys with ADD are more likely to be *hyperactive*, while girls with ADD tend to be *hyper-reactive.***

Depression and anxiety

Girls with ADD are more prone to feel depressed than guys. In fact, girls with ADD may be misdiagnosed as being only depressed, rather than having depression with ADD. (This leads to less effective treatment because the ADD gets overlooked and only the depression is treated). If you think that a lot of patterns described in the questionnaire in the front of this book describe you, and you've been diagnosed as depressed or anxious, talk to your therapist about the possibility of ADD.

PMS

Many teenage girls struggle with Premenstrual Syndrome (PMS) during the week before their menstrual period each month. They feel tense, moody, and teary—as well as experiencing physical symptoms such as bloating, fatigue, and headaches. Girls with ADD tend to experience more intense PMS symptoms than girls without ADD.

PMS symptoms are real, just like ADD is. Each tends to make the other worse. ADD patterns of forgetfulness, impatience, disorganization, and distractibility may be worse during PMS week. PMS symptoms of moodiness and overreactivity seem to be worse in girls with ADD. So . . . you need treatment for both. You need to see a doctor who is aware of ADD and PMS issues in teenage girls.

If you have difficult PMS, you should ask your gynecologist about getting treatment. Studies show that certain antidepressants can be helpful in reducing PMS.

ADD patterns in girls may be different than for guys

Many more boys than girls have been studied in ADD research. Unfortunately, since we know more about ADD in guys, they are more likely to be identified and diagnosed. Guys are more "out there" with their ADD—more hyperactive, more impulsive, more rebellious, and more likely to get angry instead of depressed. Some girls are hyperactive and impulsive like guys with ADD, but most girls with ADD are likely to be:

- Disorganized
- Forgetful
- Distractible
- Talkative
- Moody, emotional

Sadly, a lot of very smart girls with ADD are dismissed as silly, spacey, or just not very smart. Getting diagnosed and treated is important. With treatment you can get focused and use your smarts!

Social issues for girls with ADD

Many more girls than guys with ADD say that they feel badly about themselves during their high school years. Girls are more likely to feel self-conscious about being "different" than other girls. They may feel that they are too loud, too aggressive, get in trouble too much—if they have the hyperactive type of ADD.

A girl with non-hyperactive ADD may feel self-conscious, shy, and socially out of it. She may not notice things that most other girls notice. She may feel unable to keep up with the fast talk and high-activity level of other girls who don't have ADD. Either way, girls with ADD need support and reassurance. A good place to get that support is by being in a support group with other teenage girls with ADD.

GIRLS WITH ADD

Why is there a difference between girls and guys with ADD?

Probably, because a lot of ADD traits, such as not liking school, being messy, being energetic or hyper, taking risks, being argumentative, and being impulsive, are seen more as "guy" things. In fact, guys with ADD are sometimes leaders of their social group. They're the ones with the wild and crazy ideas; the ones who want to stay up all night; who may talk non-stop; take risks and stand up for their rights against teachers and parents. Of course, this is not true of ALL guys with ADD, but these patterns are much more common in guys, and many of these kinds of things are admired by other guys.

For girls, however, it's a different story. Girls are expected to be much more tuned in to people—to things that people say and don't say, to expressions on their faces. Girls are expected to be in better control, to be more neat and organized, to be well-groomed.

Sometimes quiet, inattentive girls with ADD in high school can feel overwhelmed by all of the social interaction between other girls. High school can feel much too stimulating.

Girls with ADD of the hyperactive/impulsive type have different types of social problems. They often receive much more criticism than boys for their messiness, their poor school work, and their rebellious or risky behavior. ADD behavior acceptable in guys is not so acceptable in girls.

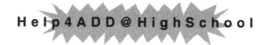

Conflicts with parents

Studies show that mothers of girls with ADD are more critical than mothers of boys with ADD. We're not sure why. It may be that girls are just expected to be more controlled and ladylike. A lot of ADD behavior is considered almost typically "boy behavior."

Mothers usually expect their sons to be less neat, less obedient, less quiet, and less academically oriented. This places an extra hard burden on girls with ADD. If you feel that you're caught in a pattern of blame and criticism with your mother, it could really help both of you to talk to your counselor together.

If your mother understands your ADD better, and if the counselor can make her more aware that mothers tend to overcriticize their daughters with ADD, then maybe this pattern can begin to change. This is important. Don't ignore this issue if you're feeling picked on at home. Constant criticism is one of the most damaging things about having ADD.

Feeling ashamed

Girls with ADD, who are adventuresome, rebellious, or impulsive during high school years, usually struggle with feelings of shame when they are a little older. Guys rarely feel this. It is related to the "boys will be boys" attitude. For most people in our society, it's much more acceptable if boys are sexually active, drink, and rebel. Parents don't like this behavior in boys, but they are less angry than when a daughter behaves in this way. Sadly, girls who are blamed and criticized by parents and teachers, often grow up to condemn themselves.

GIRLS WITH ADD

What can you do? Give yourself a break! Don't join the chorus of voices which criticize you. Self-control is just as hard for you as it is for guys. As you grow up, you will get better at stopping to think before you act. The goal is to learn how to function better in the future without condemning yourself for what has happened in the past.

Strengths for Girls with ADD

Girls with ADD have real strengths that help them cope with ADD better. Girls are usually better at verbal expression and understanding and expressing their feelings. This means that they are more likely to be helped by counseling and coaching.

Girls are often better at looking at themselves accurately, and understanding why they do things—making it much easier to think about their problems and find solutions.

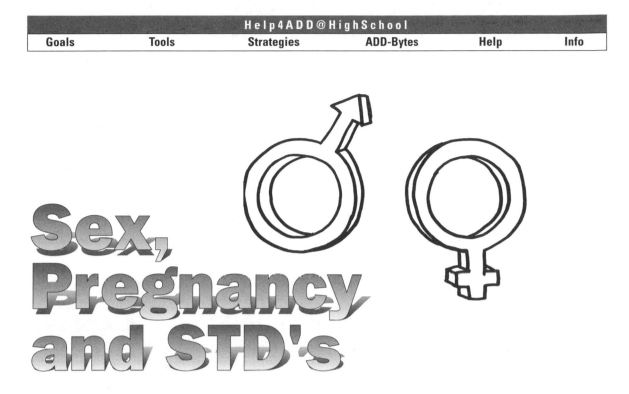

Sex, Pregnancy and STD's

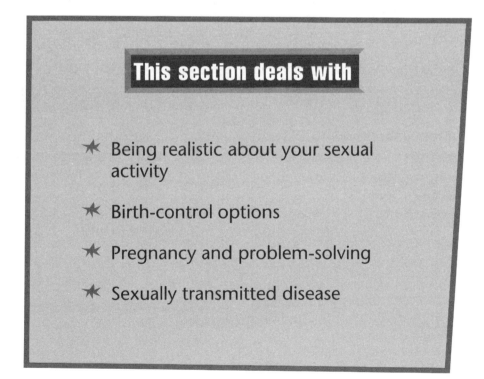

This section deals with

* Being realistic about your sexual activity

* Birth-control options

* Pregnancy and problem-solving

* Sexually transmitted disease

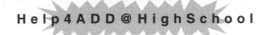
Being realistic about your sexual activity

Teens with ADD are more likely to take risks and be more impulsive than their peers. The price for taking sexual risks can be high—an unwanted pregnancy or a sexually transmitted disease.

If you are already sexually active, or are thinking of becoming sexually active, then you need to be informed about birth control and sexually transmitted diseases, or "STDs."

Your parents, if like many other parents, are not prepared for you to become sexually active in high school. Some parents, even if they know that their daughter is sexually active, refuse to condone her sexual activity by helping her to obtain birth-control pills. Parents of sons in high school often "look the other way," and don't talk frankly about pregnancy risks and sexually transmitted diseases.

Whether or not your parents are comfortable with the issue of your sexuality during high school, they need to understand, and *you* need to understand that:

> **Teen sex may be a problem, but teen pregnancy is a much bigger problem.**

Both teenagers with ADD and their parents are often prone to ignore the problem because it may feel too uncomfortable to face. But ignoring the problem can lead to very painful results for everyone in the family.

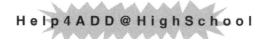

Birth-control options

If you are sexually active you need good birth control.

The Pill

One of the most effective forms of birth control is the pill. However, if you are absent-minded and forget to take it on a daily basis for 21 days during each menstrual cycle, then you run the risk of becoming pregnant.

Condoms

Condoms are much less reliable than the pill. They can tear or come off during sex. But they are much better than nothing at all. If you are a girl with ADD, don't let a boy talk you out of using a condom during sex. You're the one taking the risk of pregnancy! Even if you use other birth control, condoms are important for safe sex.

Spermicides

Spermicides are types of creams or jellies that a girl puts inside her vagina before sex to kill the sperm that might make her pregnant. Spermicides and condoms can work pretty well when used together, but few teens go around with condoms and spermicide jelly "just in case."

Diaphragms

A diaphragm is a flexible ring, covered with a thin sheet of rubberized material that a female places inside her vagina to help prevent sperm from entering her uterus to make her pregnant. They should be used with a spermicidal jelly to be effective.

Injections

Girls can have birth-control shots that are effective for several months. These may be a good choice, especially for girls who are forgetful and inconsistent about using birth control.

Pregnancy and problem-solving

ADD and Birth Control

The biggest birth-control issue for most teens with ADD is

consistency.

Because many teens with ADD are impulsive and forgetful, they typically become pregnant through inconsistent birth-control use.

Studies show that girls with ADD are more likely to become pregnant than other high school girls. It is also probably true that boys with ADD are more likely to get their girlfriend pregnant than boys without ADD.

Why? Because high school students with ADD tend to be impulsive and have sex on the spur of the moment without taking birth-control precautions.

Fact:

The percentage of adopted children with ADD is much higher than non-adopted children.

Why? Probably because of pregnancy among teens with ADD. These are the teens who are at greater risk of becoming pregnant, and are not prepared to become parents. Their babies, born with ADD, are adopted by other families.

What can you do to prevent pregnancy?

❶ Be aware of the risk.

❷ If you feel you can't talk to your parents about needing birth control, look for another adult who can help.

❸ Avoid situations that will damage your judgment— such as drinking or taking drugs with your boyfriend or girlfriend.

❹ Always have a condom with you if you are sexually active. Although condoms aren't the safest form of birth control, they are much better than nothing.

❺ Seek counseling to help you talk realistically with your parent about birth control. More and more high school students are sexually active, but many parents are unable to accept this and deal with it appropriately.

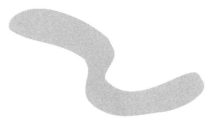

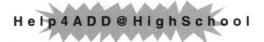

Sexually transmitted diseases

Very few teenagers want to think about the possibility of getting a sexually transmitted disease (STD). Unfortunately, they often deal with their discomfort by pretending that there is nothing to worry about.

Teenagers with ADD are at greater risk for contracting an STD. Out of impulsivity, they may drink too much and then have sex with someone they don't know well, but don't think of the consequences.

Some sexually transmitted diseases can be treated easily by a doctor. The only price is the discomfort or embarrassment of getting treatment. Others, however, are incurable.

Herpes

Herpes is a lifelong, incurable condition, which is periodically "active." Once you have herpes, you will need to inform your sexual partners for the rest of your life that you have herpes. Even after you are in a stable relationship or marriage, you will need to be careful about your condition and to not have sexual contact when your herpes is active. Casual, impulsive sex is not worth a lifetime of herpes.

HIV

The most dangerous sexually transmitted disease is HIV or AIDS. Everyone has heard of it, but most teenagers believe that only gay men or intravenous drug users are at risk. This is not true. There are many students with HIV on college campuses, and in high school. HIV can be in your body for a long time without causing symptoms. The only way to know is to have a blood test. HIV may not even show up in a blood test for several months after exposure.

Safe Sex

The only way to be sure of not getting a sexually transmitted disease is to not have sexual contact, or to only have "safe sex." "Safe sex" means to always use a condom and to never exchange bodily fluids. If you choose to be sexually active, both you and your partner should have blood tests if you have had other sexual partners, even if that contact was weeks or months ago. Few teenagers take any of this seriously, and some of them pay for it with illness, and even death. Don't let anyone embarass you or tell you it's silly. *Always* use condoms. It can save your life!

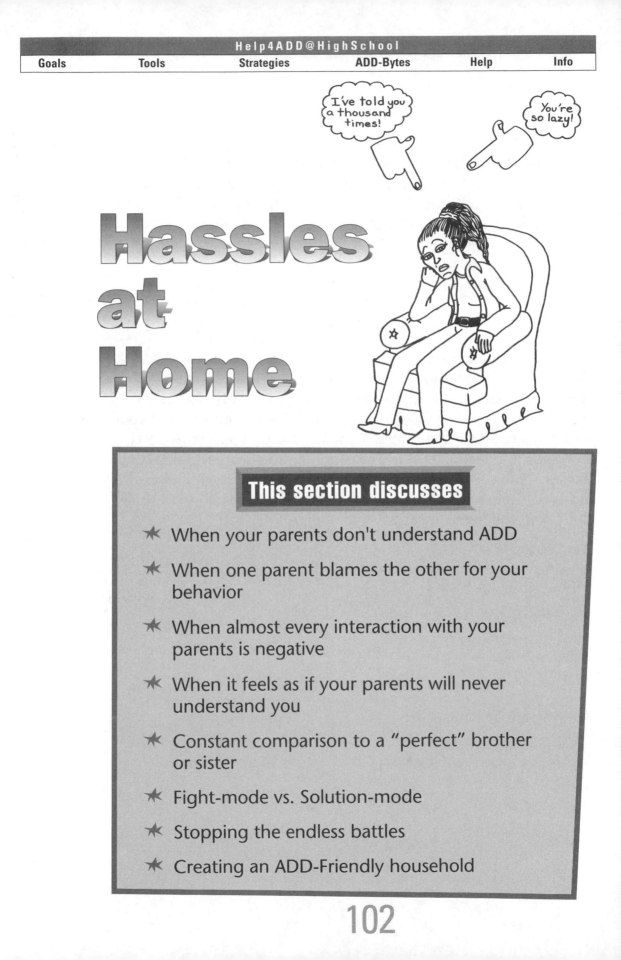

Hassles at Home

This section discusses

★ When your parents don't understand ADD

★ When one parent blames the other for your behavior

★ When almost every interaction with your parents is negative

★ When it feels as if your parents will never understand you

★ Constant comparison to a "perfect" brother or sister

★ Fight-mode vs. Solution-mode

★ Stopping the endless battles

★ Creating an ADD-Friendly household

Battles with your parents

Does your home feel like a battleground? Unfortunately this happens in many families of teens with ADD. Even without ADD the teenage years can be difficult. But ADD can make family battles more frequent and intense.

Not every family with an ADD teen needs counseling, but if your family seems "stuck"—can't talk together, find common ground, enjoy each other's company, or constructively try to solve problems, then family therapy with an ADD specialist may help.

When your mother or father doesn't understand ADD

Sometimes problems with ADD can be worse because your parents don't understand how you are affected by ADD. They may get angry at you for something you have done unintentionally— like forgetting a book at school that you needed for homework. They may get angry because they don't believe you are "really trying."

> *Chris' father seemed constantly annoyed at Chris. Mr. Knowles was a retired Navy officer who worked as an engineer. He was a very organized, precise man, who was frequently upset by Chris' forgetfulness and lack of organization. When Chris discovered that he needed a book or special materials at the last minute for a school project, his father refused to take him to get them. Mr. Knowles repeatedly said, "That's the only way you'll learn." Mr. Knowles knew that his son was diagnosed with ADD, but had learned very little about it. He believed that Chris' forgetfulness was due to lack of motivation.*

It was helpful for Mr. Knowles to talk to a counselor alone, to hear about other families with ADD teenagers, and to do some reading about ADD. Chris' father was an intelligent man. When he read about the scientific evidence for ADD, and explanations about neurochemicals and frontal-lobe functioning, he decided that ADD wasn't just some psycho-babble theory. He also inter-acted with adult men with ADD in the local ADD support group. Chris' father became convinced that Chris wasn't just being "im-mature," and began to seek ways to help Chris become more focused and organized.

HASSLES AT HOME

When one parent blames the other for your behavior

Your parents may repeatedly fight over you. One of your parents may believe that the other makes excuses for you, or isn't strict enough. In many families parents end up at opposite poles. One of your parents may overprotect you. The other parent may be so frustrated or angry with you that his/her mind is closed to the difficulties caused by ADD.

> In Brian's family, this was the case. Brian's father had been raised as an only child by a stay-at-home mother who took care of everything for him. Brian's father wanted his son to enjoy the same carefree childhood that he had.
>
> Brian rarely helped out around the house, despite the fact that he was the oldest and his mother worked full-time. His mother, however, resented Brian's self-centered, inconsiderate approach to life. She felt that he needed to learn to take care of himself, and not to expect everything to be done for him. She and her husband had repeated fights over what was reasonable to expect from Brian.

Brian's family reached a different sort of solution. Even with counseling, his mother could never convince his father to expect more independent functioning from him, but both parents agreed that he would do well in a boarding school where he could pursue his sports interests while getting more academic support. This removed Brian from his parents' battle over him, and placed him in an environment which expected more responsibility from him.

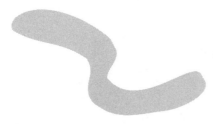

When almost every interaction at home is negative

Some teens with ADD defend themselves by intentionally annoying their parent(s). And some parents get to the point that almost everything they say is critical, angry, or negative.

In Mandy's household the fighting was constant. No one seemed to know what to do. Both of her parents worked. Whichever parent walked in the door first, tired from work and automatically upset with Mandy, usually began the fight. "Why isn't this kitchen cleaned up? No, you can't have the car. You've got homework to do." Mandy typically exploded in anger, yelling at her mother or father, slamming the door to her room, and spending the evening on the phone talking to friends about how awful her parents were, and how she couldn't wait to leave home.

Mandy's household benefitted tremendously from counseling. Both parents came to realize that their own stress levels were contributing to the daily problems. They both worked long hours and expected Mandy, as the oldest child, to take on major responsibilities for her younger sister and for the household in the afternoon. They didn't fully recognize the stress level Mandy felt coping with her ADD in high school.

Mandy arrived home exhausted, and still faced homework. The last thing she was in the mood for was to supervise her 11-year-old sister and to clean up the kitchen. Through counseling, everyone recognized the need for positive interactions, for quiet zones in the house, and for less stress. Her parents arranged their work schedules so that they alternated coming home earlier. Mandy and her mother made sure they had time to talk in the late afternoon— often cleaning up the kitchen and preparing dinner together.

Shannon, Mandy's little sister, was given the responsibility to check in with her mother or father at work, and to let them know where she would be. They no longer left Mandy in charge of Shannon—an arrangement which both of them had resented. And everyone recognized the need to problem-solve rather than criticize and argue when new problems arose.

Problem-solving and negotiating at home

Whether you go to counseling as a family, or are able to work things out at home, your goal as a family should be to shift from fight-mode to problem-solving mode. In a problem-solving mode, the game isn't "pin the blame" on the donkey. When you are in problem-solving mode, everyone in the family is working in the same direction, looking for a solution that will be best for everyone.

Does the solution-mode seem like pie-in-the-sky to you? Has your family fought for so long that you can't imagine cooperation? You may need to work with a family counselor for a while. At first your family may need to practice problem-solving in the counselor's office to get better at it. Many families are so much in the habit of blaming, defending, and fighting, that it will take a while to develop new habits.

Don't assume it's impossible. The fact that your parent bought this book, and that you're reading it, are positive signs that your family wants things to be better.

What is an ADD-Friendly household?

A household designed to avoid or minimize the chronic problems caused by ADD.

- It's a family that looks for ways to **simplify routines and solve problems.**

- It's a **home furnished in a casual, sturdy easy-to-maintain style,** where no one is in trouble for tipping their chair in the kitchen or eating snacks in the family room.

- It's a **family that focuses on the important things**—like being loving, encouraging, and cooperative. An ADD-Friendly family doesn't sweat the details—like who left the wet towel on the bathroom floor.

- It's a **family that learns to be patient** when people are short-tempered, and where people apologize sincerely when they occasionally "lose it."

- It's a **family that learns to laugh over ADD dilemmas** and goofs, and to emphasize what family members do right instead of what they do wrong.

- It has a convenient **message center** where family members can write each other notes and reminders and is located where people are sure to look.

- It's a **family where it's OK to be different** from each other and OK to be yourself.

- It's a **family where people make sure to spend time enjoying each other** rather than just focusing on problems.

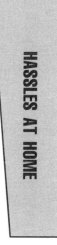

HASSLES AT HOME

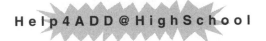
What can change your household from a battle zone to a comfort zone?

❶ Learn to problem-solve as a family.

❷ Become educated about ADD as a family.

> **An ADD-Smart family understands that ADD isn't an excuse; it's an explanation that calls for ADD-smart solutions.**

If someone forgets something repeatedly and you think it's because they just don't care, it's natural to become angry. If you think the forgetting is related to ADD, then you are more likely to look for a solution—"How can we make sure you remember this time?," rather than threatening, "The next time you forget, you're grounded for a week."

❸ Look for ways as a family to **design an ADD-Friendly household.**

> When is the last time you enjoyed spending time with each of your parents? When is the last time you really talked openly with your parents about your hopes, your fears, your frustrations? If your family isn't "ADD savvy," then you and your parents can find an endless list of issues to battle over. Going to an ADD specialist as a family may help the problem-solving process to begin. Good luck and get going! It doesn't have to be an endless battle.

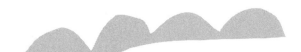

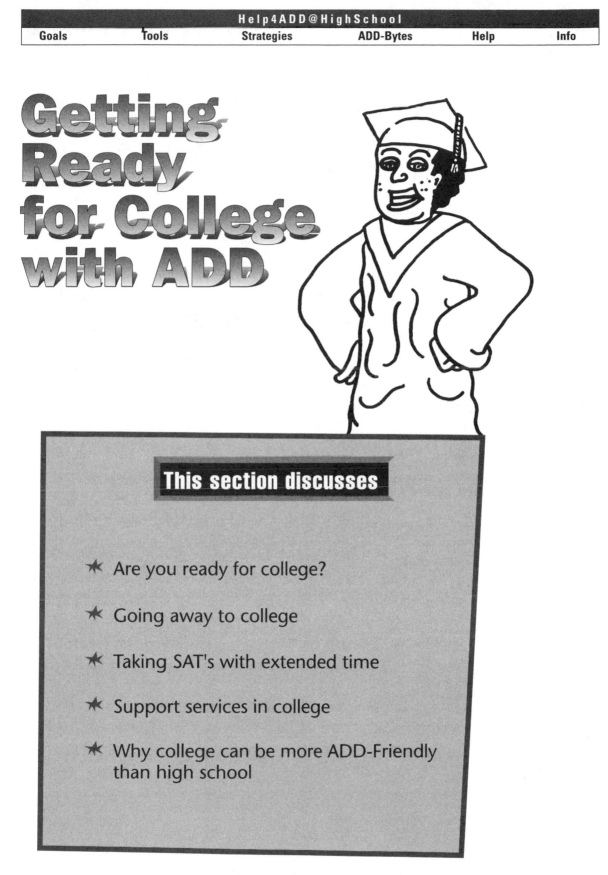

Getting Ready for College with ADD

This section discusses

★ Are you ready for college?

★ Going away to college

★ Taking SAT's with extended time

★ Support services in college

★ Why college can be more ADD-Friendly than high school

109

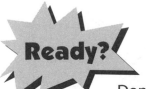

Are you ready for college?

Don't automatically assume that you should go directly to college from high school. This is a good choice for some students with ADD, but for others it's a course headed for failure.

Many students do better in college after they have been out in the world for a while. They may need a break from school if high school has been very stressful. They may need to work for a while before they can choose a career direction that motivates them.

Just because you don't go straight to college doesn't mean that you won't go later—although many parents fear this.

Be honest with yourself and with your parents. If you're not sure, you might consider your local community college for a semester or two. This is a much less-expensive venture for students who have mixed feelings about college.

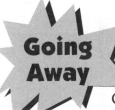

Going away to college

Going away to college can seem fun and exciting, but be sure you've chosen a school that gives you enough structure and support. A big state university may seem appealing, but it's easy to get lost in the crowd. Classes for freshman are huge, you have little or no contact with professors.

Often smaller colleges with good ADD/LD support services are a better choice—especially in your first two years of college.

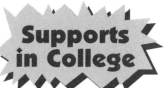

Supports for ADD and LD

Don't make the mistake of deciding in advance that you don't want any supports for your ADD. It's not at all like LD or ADD supports in high school. You will not ever be singled out or embarrassed. You will not be placed in a special program, unless you specifically apply for a special program.

There is no negative image attached to LD or ADD supports in college—the services are there for your benefit. Take full advantage of them. They can make a big difference in your chances for success.

You should be aware that all colleges don't have the same quality of support services. Choose your college very carefully. In the resource section at the back of this book you will find books on surviving in college with ADD. These can be very helpful to you when you are ready to begin visiting colleges.

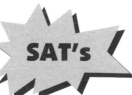

Taking the SAT's with extended time

Many college counselors will advise you to take the Scholastic Assessment Test (SAT) in a standard format, and then decide whether you want to take them untimed.

This is because most counselors assume that it's better to apply to college without indicating that you have ADD or a learning disability.

Do you really want to go to a college that has a negative attitude toward students with ADD or LD?

It seems that a more successful approach is to take your SAT's untimed, earn the highest score you can, and then look for the best school you can find that has very good supports for students with ADD.

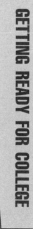

GETTING READY FOR COLLEGE

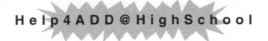

Why College is more ADD-Friendly

Many students with ADD find that college is much better than high school.

Bigger variety of colleges

Most high schools are pretty much alike, unless you attend a private school. In college however, there is a huge range of choices—community colleges; small private colleges; large state universities; colleges which let you design your own course of study; colleges in which you take only one course at a time; colleges on the quarter system; or on the semester system; colleges that offer night courses for students who work; and colleges which specialize in your area of interest. With all of these choices, you have a better chance of choosing a college which will be a good match for your needs and interests.

Wider choice of courses

Colleges all have requirements, but you have a much wider range of choices when selecting your courses.

Fewer class hours

Sitting in class for hours on end is very difficult for most students with ADD. In college, you are normally in class for only two-to-four hours each day, and may have some days with no classes at all.

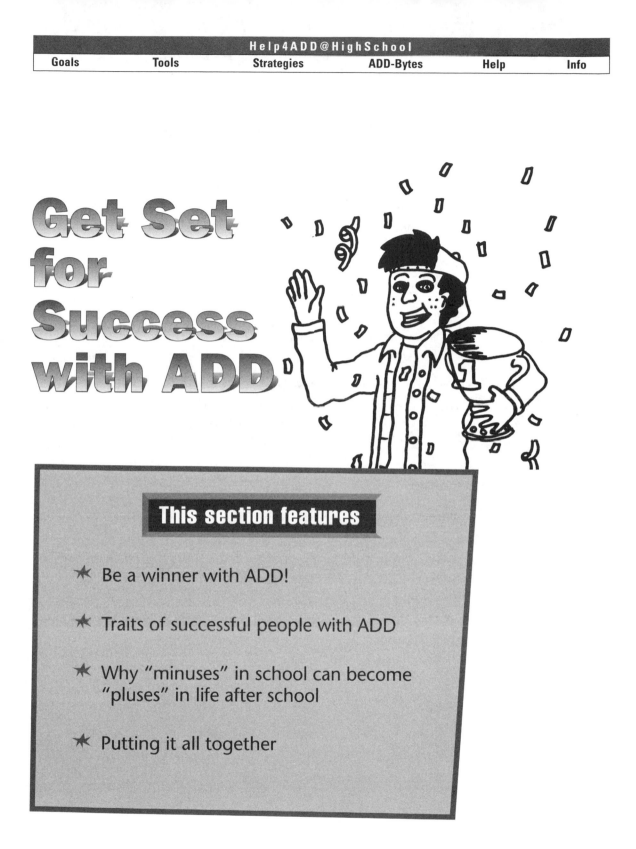

Get Set for Success with ADD

This section features

★ Be a winner with ADD!

★ Traits of successful people with ADD

★ Why "minuses" in school can become "pluses" in life after school

★ Putting it all together

Be a winner with ADD!

You were born with ADD and it will influence you all your life. But not all of the influences are problems! There are positive ADD traits not just negative ones. By understanding exactly how you are affected—you can take advantage of your "ADD pluses" and learn how to take charge of your "ADD minuses."

ADD "pluses" are terrific—like having a lot of energy, having tons of ideas, being creative, noticing things no one else does, and being enthusiastic. Many people with ADD are huge successes in life—in politics, in the entertainment field, in sports, in sales, in business, in computers, and in lots of other fields.

People who are successes with ADD are the ones who learned how to take charge of their ADD, and found just the right spot to take advantage of their strengths. That's what this book is designed to help you do! By reading this book, and putting into action what is recommended, it will put you on the road to becoming an ADD success in life!

Traits of Successful people with ADD

A professor named Paul Gerber studied highly successful people with learning disabilities to see what they had in common. Many of the things he learned can apply to people with ADD.   Dr. Gerber's list of success traits is listed on the next page, and we've added a couple of extra ones that are special for ADD.

Internal

Internal Success Factors

- ◆ Strong motivation
- ◆ Determination—stick-to-it-iveness
- ◆ A need to control your own life and your future
- ◆ Ability to see your ADD and/or LD in a positive light
- ◆ Planfulness and being goal-oriented
- ◆ Independence, while seeking help when you need it

External

External Success Factors

- ◆ A mentor—someone who can be a model and guide for you
- ◆ Positive, supportive people around you
- ◆ Opportunities to develop new skills
- ◆ Having help available when you need it
- ◆ Having a good match between what you're good at and what you're expected to do

Some of these success traits you may already possess. Others you may need to develop with the help of counselors and coaches.

But most of all, remember that:

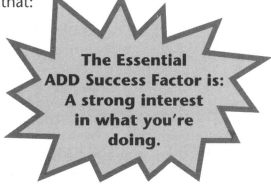

The Essential
ADD Success Factor is:
A strong interest
in what you're
doing.

A "minus" in school may be a "plus" in real life!

What is a "minus," and what is a "plus," depends on where you are. One of the wonderful things you'll discover is that lots of things that make high school hard can become real assets if you put yourself in the right place!

Let's make a list of some "ADD-minuses" and think about how they might also be "pluses."

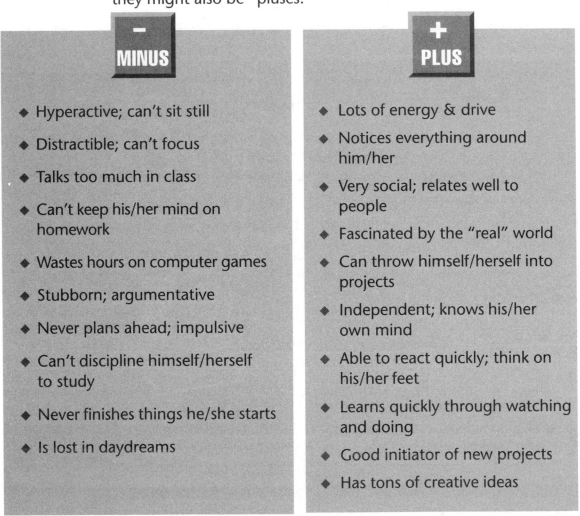

– MINUS

- ◆ Hyperactive; can't sit still
- ◆ Distractible; can't focus
- ◆ Talks too much in class
- ◆ Can't keep his/her mind on homework
- ◆ Wastes hours on computer games
- ◆ Stubborn; argumentative
- ◆ Never plans ahead; impulsive
- ◆ Can't discipline himself/herself to study
- ◆ Never finishes things he/she starts
- ◆ Is lost in daydreams

+ PLUS

- ◆ Lots of energy & drive
- ◆ Notices everything around him/her
- ◆ Very social; relates well to people
- ◆ Fascinated by the "real" world
- ◆ Can throw himself/herself into projects
- ◆ Independent; knows his/her own mind
- ◆ Able to react quickly; think on his/her feet
- ◆ Learns quickly through watching and doing
- ◆ Good initiator of new projects
- ◆ Has tons of creative ideas

High school may not be the best place to take advantage of your ADD "pluses." After high school, you can make choices to really take advantage of them.

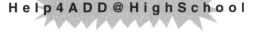

GET SET FOR SUCCESS

Putting it all together

We have covered many topics in Help4ADD@HighSchool. It may seem a little overwhelming right now, but if you identify the areas that are most important for you to work on and tackle them one at a time, you'll find yourself taking charge of your ADD and feeling much more positive about your future.

❶ Don't try to tackle this on your own.

It's hard to stay on track while you try to learn better ways to study, plan, organize, and problem-solve. You'll make more progress if you work with a tutor, counselor, or coach, who can help you set goals and keep on track.

❷ Think about ALL of you, not just school.

If you are struggling with bad feelings about yourself, are having problems with friends, or find yourself feeling anxious, depressed, and overwhelmed much of the time, don't ignore it. These are all treatable problems. You may need counseling and possibly medication in order to feel and function better. This doesn't mean that you'll always need therapy, but high school can be very tough for a teen with ADD.

❸ Get your parents on your side.

If your parents are usually annoyed, nagging, and negative toward you, then you could benefit by having your parents come to counseling with you sometimes. That way you can decide as a family how to deal with family conflict, rules, restrictions, homework, privileges, and expectations.   If you're all on the same team, things will be better for the whole family.

❹ Look toward the future—the best is yet to come.

Your high school years may be some of the toughest years you'll have. If you work hard to take charge of your ADD, there are many choices and opportunities waiting for you after high school.

117

Teen ADD Resources

Teenagers with ADD: A Parent's Guide by Chris Dendy.

Give Your ADD Teen a Chance by Lynn Weiss.

ADHD & Teens: A Parent's Guide to Making It Through the Tough Years by Colleen Alexander-Roberts.

ADD and Adolescence: Strategies for Success from CHADD

Get Out of My Life, But first, Could You Drive Me and Cheryl to the Mall? Anthony E. Wolf, Ph.D.

Adolescents and ADD: Gaining the Advantage by Patricia O. Quinn, M.D.

TEEN ADD RESOURCES

High School seniors! Look for Kathleen Nadeau's next book called,

Ready, Set, Go!

Successful transition to independence
for teens and young adults with ADD

Ready, Set, Go! will focus on many practical issues to help you prepare for successful independence—whether you go away to college or go to work.

- Making ADD-Friendly college choices

- Training alternatives to college

- Making ADD-Friendly career choices

- Gaining your independence one step at a time

- Building a partnership with your parents

- Dealing with roommates and ADD

- Managing your money

- Life-Management Skills

- Learning on-the-job social skills

- Job interviews; resume writing

- Finding and keeping a job

- Planning for the future

Look for *Ready, Set, Go!* in 1999 from Advantage Books.

ALSO AVAILABLE FROM
ADVANTAGE BOOKS

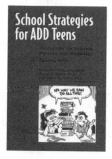

School Strategies for ADD Teens
by Kathleen Nadeau, Ellen Dixon, & Sue Biggs

This well-organized book outlines how to get the help you need in high school for your AD/HD.

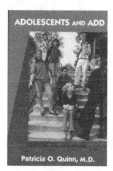

Adolescents and ADD
by Patricia O. Quinn, M.D.

Written for students with ADD as they enter middle or high school and filled with valuable advice from doctors, teachers, and other students with ADD, who have experienced the same fears, successes, and disappointments. Provides tips on getting organized, achieving greater success, and how to become your own advocate.

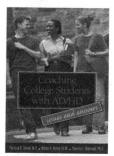

Coaching College Students with ADHD
by Patricia Quinn, Nancy Ratey, and Theresa Maitland

A must for all coaches and college service providers, as well as students with ADHD. Provides answers to those difficult issues   that students must face on a daily basis.

Understanding Girls with AD/HD
by K. Nadeau, P. Quinn, E. Littman

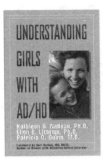

Understanding Girls with AD/HD is a ground-breaking book for parents, health care professionals and educators, designed to increase awareness of girls with AD/HD, many of whom continue to remain unidentified. Dealing with developmental issues from preschool through high school. it gives the older girl with ADHD the information she needs to begin to cope with her ADHD in a more mature fashion.

College Survival Guide for ADD and LD Students
by Kathleen G. Nadeau, Ph.D.

Don't plan for college without this! This manual outlines the entire process, including college selection, assessing services on campus, academic counseling, selection of a major, study tips, as well as a long section on typical problems and ways to overcome them.

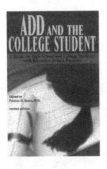

ADD and the College Student
by Patricia O. Quinn, M.D.

This handbook for high school juniors and seniors as well as college students with ADD contains information on ADD and its impact on college life. Packed with practical advice and strategies, it will help students with ADD effectively navigate the difficult transition from high school to college.

I would like to order the following books:

Quantity	Book Title	Price
_____	ADD-Friendly High Schools A Guide For Parents, Teachers and Administrators	$14.95
_____	Coaching College Students	$12.95
_____	Adolescents and ADD	$12.95
_____	ADD and the College Student	$14.95
_____	College Survival Guide for ADD and LD Students	$9.95
_____	Understanding Girls with ADHD	$19.95

Shipping/ Handling: $4 for 1st book and $1.75 each additional

MD residents add 5% sales tax   TOTAL ORDER $_____

Order now using the form below
call 1-888-238-8588 or
visit our website at www.addvance.com

Name
Address
City   State   Zip
Credit Card   Exp Date
Signature

Make checks payable to: **ADVANTAGE BOOKS**
                          8607 Cedar St.
                          Silver Spring, MD 20910

Call for bulk rates and discounts for orders of 10 or more books